STILL HOT!

STILL HOT!

42 brilliantly honest menopause stories

KAYE ADAMS
& VICKY ALLAN

BLACK & WHITE PUBLISHING

First published 2020
by Black & White Publishing Ltd
Nautical House, 104 Commercial Street
Edinburgh, EH6 6NF

1 3 5 7 9 10 8 6 4 2   20 21 22 23

ISBN: 978 1 78530 310 4

This book is a work of non-fiction, based on interviews about the lives, experiences and
recollections of its contributors. The authors have stated to the publishers that the contents of
this book are true to the best of their knowledge.

All photos are reproduced courtesy of individual authors except those otherwise credited.
The publisher has made every reasonable effort to contact copyright holders of images in this book.
Any errors are inadvertent and anyone who for any reason has not been contacted is invited to write
to the publisher so that a full acknowledgment can be made in subsequent editions of this work.

The views expressed by the authors and contributors in this book are their personal views.
Any comments or views regarding medical matters are the authors' and contributors' own
and are not intended as, and do not constitute, medical advice. Neither the authors nor the
publisher can accept any responsibility for anything relating to such views, or any consequences
thereof, that occur either directly or indirectly from the contents of this book.

A CIP catalogue record for this book is available from the British Library.

Typeset by Iolaire, Newtonmore
Printed and bound by CPI Group (UK) Ltd, Croydon, CR0 4YY

Love and gratitude to those who came before.
Love and fortitude to those about to go there.

Still Hot! all began as a chat between the two of us in a café. Now here it is, a great chorus of voices, all telling this diverse story of the menopause. Thanks for joining us. Let's keep the chorus going.

Kaye & Vicky

STILL

(adv)

Up to and including the present; even now;
nevertheless, all the same.

HOT

(adj)

Having a high temperature; performed with skill
and daring and energy; full of passion or other strong
emotions; currently in demand; lusty and desirable.

Contents

Out of the Menopausal Closet
Kaye Adams......1

They spoke, we listened......5

RAGE

Felicity Everett......9

Louise Newson......16

Julie Graham......25

India Gary-Martin......35

FOG

Pippa Marriott......43

Sayeeda Warsi......50

Angie Greaves......60

GRIEF

Andrea Macfarlane......71

Sahira Ahmad Belcher......80

Yvonne John......86

Xinran Xue......94

Shalini Bhalla-Lucas......103

LOW

Denise Welch...... 111   Lorraine Kelly...... 121

Helen FitzGerald...... 131

STRONGER

Erica Clarkson...... 141   Louise Minchin...... 156

Melissa Wall...... 164

SPARK

Trinny Woodall...... 171   Anthea Turner...... 179

Shahzadi Harper...... 188   Tania Glyde...... 197

PAIN

Jane Lewis...... 211   Alison Martin-Campbell...... 220

Michelle Heaton...... 229

DESIRE

Tracey Cox...... 241   Penny Pepper...... 251

Nimmy March...... 256   Marie Louise Cochrane...... 261

BREEZE

Carol Smillie...... 271   Val McDermid...... 277

Yasmin Alibhai-Brown...... 281   Pinky Lilani...... 286

FREEDOM

Miranda Sawyer......291

Kirsty Wark......302

Bunny Cook......309

Danusia Malina-Derben......318

Sharmila Mehta......326

Paulette Edwards......333

WISDOM

Sharon Blackie......341

Jody Day......355

Susie Orbach......367

Sharing, the Menopause Revolution
Vicky Allan......373

Resources & Reading......381

Menopause Bingo......385

Thanks......387

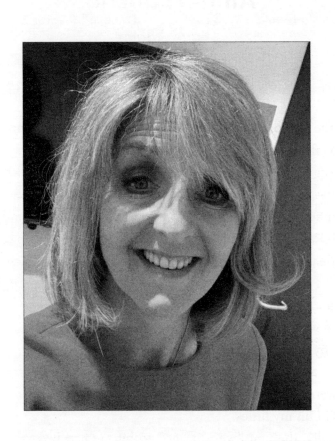

Out of the Menopausal Closet
An Introduction

Kaye Adams

It was the stuff of madness. We were at Heathrow Airport and I could hear my flight being called. I knew Ian and the kids were waiting for me – hugely excited at the prospect of a big trip to LA – but *I just did not want to leave the toilet cubicle*. Nothing would have made me happier at that point than if the flight had been cancelled and I could GO HOME. Better still, if I could magically teleport myself there and hide under the duvet until the awful pounding in my chest went away.

I hadn't even needed the loo, I just needed to hide.

I've never been the kind of person who wanted to hide. I am pretty gobby, by nature.

Panic attacks, anxiety, that heavy weight bearing down on the chest were all alien to me.

Until I hit my fifties.

Actually, the first "weird thing" to hit me had been a couple of years earlier. Things were going well work-wise. My friend and fellow *Loose Women* panellist Nadia Sawalha and I had been given a Sunday morning show on ITV and were about to return to *Loose Women* after a longish break. My radio show was going great guns and I had several other jobs in the offing. Home life was good and the apple of my eye had just entered the frame . . . my dog, Bea!

But, despite the apparently rosy picture, inexplicably, I felt desperately low in a way I had never experienced before. Depression was once described to me as "an absence of joy" and that is exactly how it was for four, very flat months. Good things were happening, and objectively, I could see they were "good", but I got no kick from them whatsoever.

It was as if I had lost the ability to lift my spirits. When I pushed the "joy button", nothing happened and I had no idea why. That it might be connected in some way to the approaching menopause didn't even occur to me despite the fact that my periods were becoming more irregular and out-of-whack. To be absolutely honest, the menopause wasn't even on my radar.

Eventually, the clouds cleared. I breathed a sigh of relief and carried on.

And this is where I have to confess... again, something I only realised in hindsight... that I was (and probably still am) a menopause denier. The word held such negative connotations for me; of a woman who was "past her best", "over-ripe", "surplus to requirements", "irrelevant".

Despite having a very open relationship with my mum, she never ever discussed the menopause with me and I was never aware of her going through it. She was also incredibly secretive about her age; she once ended up in a police station for refusing to give her date of birth when she was pulled over for speeding. It clearly rubbed off on me. Deep in my psyche must linger a belief that getting older is a negative thing and the menopause is proof positive of ageing so...

Deny, deny, deny.

It's pathetic really. Who was I trying to kid? I recall being on a skiing holiday with a group of women, perhaps just a couple of years older than me. One night at dinner, in the classic alpine chalet, I struggled to disguise my horror as they all sat fanning themselves with the menus and blowing down their necklines. "That will *never* be me," I vowed.

Deny, deny, deny.

As buttoned up as I was about the menopause, Ms Sawalha was open and honest. She freely described the mood swings, the skin itchiness, the insomnia and the all-round rubbishness of the menopause while I drove her to complete and utter distraction by claiming it wasn't happening to me and that she was being melodramatic as usual. It was largely all in jest, but I could tell she wanted to throttle me at times. "You are PERI!" (as in perimenopausal), she would scream at me, in frustration. Maybe, but I wasn't going to admit it. The reality was that I didn't have any of the classic menopausal symptoms that tend to get discussed. I never had hot flushes and therefore never had the need to fan myself with the menu and blow down my chest. I didn't suffer from insomnia or achy bones or dry skin or hair loss. I did get a mild version of what I now know to be night sweats but I would simply stick my leg out from under the duvet for some cool air and snooze on. The unfamiliar panic attacks and feelings of anxiety, I pushed to one side.

I hope I did manage to be sympathetic towards Nadia and all the other friends that I spent many hours with, listening to their menopause symptoms. I hope I *ooh*ed and *aah*ed in all the right places, despite seldom sharing much of my own experience. In truth, I think that by constantly putting a lid on my emotions and refusing to acknowledge what was happening, I was actually the biggest loser.

My early fifties were hellish years. My beloved dad became very ill after getting close to eighty while enjoying rude health. From then until his death two and a half years later, he required full-time care. Shortly after Dad died, my fabulous and formidable mum had a stroke from which she never recovered in any great sense and she died eighteen months later. I had no difficulty in accounting for my tight chest, tight throat and short fuse. Watching them slip away felt like four years of failure and loss, never quite feeling I was doing enough, either for my parents or my teenage children.

At work, I just kept on keeping on, trying not to drop the ball.

Maybe Mum did me a favour passing on her menopause denial, because I just didn't have time or headspace for it, or so I thought.

In retrospect, I honestly wish I had taken that time and headspace to acknowledge that my body was going through enormous change, that my hormones were all over the place and that there were reasons for me feeling so lost beyond the painful circumstances I found myself in. I might have been kinder to myself. I might have let myself ask for help instead of soldiering on . . . in denial.

Sticking your fingers in your ears and chanting *la-la-la* is rarely an effective strategy in adult life, but it is remarkable how transformational it can be just to share experiences and to remind ourselves that we are part of a tribe as well as unique.

And, with that in mind, this frank, funny (and only slightly grumpy) book shares the experiences of forty-two fabulous human beings who have all been through the menopause . . . in their own way.

I am proud to be one of them.

Still Hot! is my coming out . . . as a menopausal woman.

4

They spoke, we listened

Still Hot! is a collection brought together in a spirit of inclusivity. There are stories here from heterosexual, white women, from people of colour, from nonbinary and trans people, from the childless and the childfree, those early to the change, those late, those catapulted there by surgery, all of whom have gone through or are going through the perimenopause or menopause.

Each person in these pages tells their own story in their own way and using the words they feel comfortable with. Those words were generally given as spoken interviews and edited and brought together here. We know it can be hard to put such personal stories out there – and we respect and value their bravery in doing it.

It should also be noted that the solutions each individual has found in their experiences of the menopause may not work for everyone, or even long term for themselves. This is not a guide on how to deal with symptoms, but a sharing of stories, a book of solidarity and taboo-busting. If you are struggling with symptoms and want help, we advise you first visit your GP. For more information, you may also want to look up some of the resources, books and websites detailed at the back of *Still Hot!*.

What even is the "menopause"?

The menopause is considered to be the time when an individual stops having periods and is no longer able to conceive "naturally".

There is some fluidity around the terms "perimenopause", "menopause" and "postmenopause" and contributors may use these words differently, according to their own experiences and understanding. These broad definitions might be helpful.

Perimenopause refers to the eight to ten years before menopause when the ovaries slowly produce less oestrogen.

Menopause refers to the time when menstrual periods have stopped for at least a year.

Postmenopause is the stage of life after the last period was twelve months ago or longer.

RAGE

(noun)

Ferocious, uncontrollable anger, which surfaces
seemingly from nowhere and in response to even the
smallest trigger.

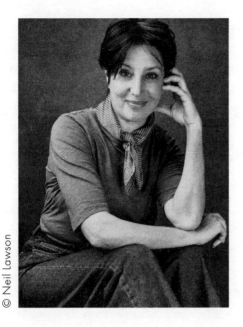

Felicity Everett

Author

"You're not seriously suggesting we put the telly there?"

Felicity Everett, 59, is the bestselling author of *The Story of Us*, *The Move* and *The People at Number 9*. She has four children and a grandchild. When she and her husband moved to an idyllic cottage in the Cotswolds to start a new life, with an almost empty nest, her menopause symptoms started to emerge.

~

My poor husband. He was doing something relatively innocent, plugging the aerial into the telly in the living room when this rage surged through me.

I think it was partly to do with territory. We had moved to a new home, an idyllic little cottage in the Cotswolds. He had just retired. Before that, he'd been at work all day and the home was where I stayed and worked and it felt almost like I'd sprayed in the corners and here he was coming in and taking over. I got blind rage about it.

"You're not seriously suggesting we put the telly there?" I said.

He did absolutely get it in the neck.

I felt as though what little area of influence and decision-making I had was being taken away from me. I suppose I felt powerless.

I didn't understand what that rage was. I can't even remember if I thought it was hormonal at the time. It went away, but the feeling of upset and anger didn't quite because I think I felt I was being blamed for something. It was mixed up with other things that we were addressing in a long marriage.

I'd had perimenopausal symptoms before that. When we were living in Australia for a few years previous to it, my periods had been sporadic but with massive flooding. There were a couple of embarrassing situations where I wasn't expecting it. I don't remember mood swings back then. It was just periods going berserk and coming and going.

The whole thing has been very hard to unpick for me because after twenty-five years of my life being very steady, living in one place, in London, with the same people around, raising a family, suddenly we then had ten years of upheaval, in which we first moved to Australia and then back here to the Cotswolds. My family was also growing up and leaving home and it coincided with all of that – as it so often does.

Our old home in London had in some way represented everything I thought I was – a mum, a writer, a friend and neighbour. I had been very sociable and suddenly all of that was stripped away.

There was also an awful lot of life-event stuff that really muddied the waters. My husband took early retirement. We were there together in this quite small cottage. We didn't know anybody. Our youngest daughter was with us. She was initially a bit disgruntled at being moved round the world willy-nilly – but then, in a flash, she was gone to uni. And that was it – quite an abrupt end to that phase of our lives. Suddenly me and my husband were left looking at each other in this strange place where we didn't know anyone.

That was when I started having massive mood swings. They felt very physical and reminded me, more than anything, of how I'd felt when I was breastfeeding. It felt that hormonal. I felt that little in charge of it. It was like the let-down reflex where I used to get this feeling of premonition, then the milk would come down and it tingled, and I would think, Oh, that's what that was.

> I could be out for a walk and it would almost feel like a truck was coming around the corner, rumbling.

With these menopause mood swings, I would get this kind of sudden feeling of foreboding and dread and kind of depression. Then I would get a strong feeling of nausea. I thought, that must be hormones – it's got to be because it was so bodily as well as psychological.

I could be out for a walk and it would almost feel like a truck was coming around the corner, rumbling. Of course it was just psychological. I couldn't really hear anything. But I would feel, "Oh shit, it's coming." It would be that sort of physical sense of something taking me over. It was almost like déjà vu. You suddenly get that very powerful sense that something's happened before.

I felt an overwhelming nausea and a melancholy. Sometimes I would have to stop because I felt so sick. And then it would, within five minutes, pass off again.

But I didn't think I was depressed. I knew my symptoms were to do with the menopause. I never really thought, This is a depression. I must go on antidepressants. I thought I was menopausal, I was hormonal, I was unhappy and I was sort of sporadically depressed but I never tied it up in a package of depression.

It came close to destroying my marriage. At one point I did storm off. Did I ever really think I was going to leave for good? I suppose it went through my head. But I never quite had the will to go off and be an independent person because I'd almost never been that. Also in my heart I didn't want to. He's my soul mate and he loves me. I love him too, although that wasn't front of my mind at the time. Plus, he's a brilliant dad and stuff, and he just didn't get this one thing of how I felt, but then I didn't get it either.

I never got much further than sitting in a lay-by and crying and hating him and then really hating myself just as much. I checked the tank. Is there enough to get to London? But then I thought, What am I going to do when I get there? Go and see the kids and they'll say, "Are you going to split up?"

No, my heart wasn't in it. I just didn't know what to do with myself really. In the end, I got some counselling and that helped.

The anger was very helpful creatively. I wrote a book about it, *The Move*, which I think was largely driven by rage. I think that's often the case with what I write actually. It's quite therapeutic. And it's a good way of splurging everything out. Then you read it back and go, "Oh, shit. Look what I've said."

I remember eventually I caught on that all this was menopause and started researching. I went on websites where people would be saying, "How do I get rid of this and that?" I thought, God, is that all you've got? I think I could cope with itchy legs. But this was the end of the world for me.

My poor old husband Mark was trying to understand, trying to get behind me, but you know, at the same time, whenever we talked about stuff, I felt as though he was saying it didn't count because it was my hormones. He wasn't, of course – he was trying to understand. But I sort of felt diminished by it, as though it was a label that meant that I didn't have to take it too seriously, because it's all a bit mad.

I went to my doctor and she said I had got in just in time because the other thing I didn't appreciate was that if you leave it too late to start HRT, or the particular kind that she was putting me on, you might miss the boat and the health risks outweigh the benefits. So she gave it to me, and I brought it back and gave it a try.

In the end I didn't keep going with it. I was so ambivalent, because just after I'd started it, there was quite a bit of worrying publicity. By the time I'd unpicked all of that, I'd stopped taking it. I just took fright and got rid of it. I thought, I don't want to be getting breast cancer in ten years, and thinking, I should have got on with it like my mum did.

I looked into HRT again, eighteen months later, thinking, Why should I go through this? But by the time I went back to the doctor she was saying, "You know, I'm not comfortable with you taking it now because of your age."

I felt like I'd got it wrong at every stage. On balance I regret not sticking with HRT first time round. I have a very strong hunch that oestrogen is a pacifying hormone which makes women docile, marriageable and able to produce children and tamp down their otherwise healthy rage, and then when nature's finished with us, we come out the other end. But the rage is impotent by then because we're written off in a way. You come out of it as a sort of asexual harridan.

And yet I feel in some ways the menopause is a superpower. It's quite creative. I feel much better as a postmenopausal woman than I did when I was going through perimenopause. It's seen by society as being very negative and I don't think it should be. It's powerful and should be harnessed.

The other thing is I went right off sex for a long period. Some of that may have been hormonal and some of it may have been that I was at such a low ebb. I didn't rate myself as a person, so I didn't see why anyone else should and that's not a good place to be in for, you know, having a healthy sex life. That has improved an awful lot since I've come through the other side.

I did feel a sense of loss. Not of my reproductive capacity, but at no longer being the conventional attractive nubile woman. I also mourned the process of being a mum and being surrounded by a family and a community. But on the other hand, I had done it and, therefore, I could sort of park it. I didn't exactly go, "Right, what's next?" – but after a lot of confusion and upset I've found what the next stage is and it's actually pretty good.

I think it must be a couple of years since I've had that kind of big premonition, doom-gloom-sickness thing, which I had regularly before. I don't get the rage either. If I get enraged now you can be pretty sure there's something to be enraged about. And, believe me, I get rage now about the state of the world.

What made it better? Probably a lot was circumstantial. It was coming to terms with things and getting on a better footing in my marriage. It was making friends locally and feeling a sense of belonging and starting to see what the next period of my life might look like. Whereas before I just felt I was all washed up and everything that mattered was finished.

Now I feel the world has opened up again because I've looked outwards. I also feel quite liberated and more me – less inclined to be that compliant role model, mum, partner and friend, and more bolshie in a good way. I feel like I was the Incredible Hulk bursting out of this containing garment and into myself. A bit scary, but also quite good.

Coming out the other side has coincided with having more time and more success in my writing career. That's helped in terms of self-esteem. Being seen and heard has been a big deal for me. That was part of why it was hard to come somewhere small and remote.

But writing books that are quite angry and exploring things I'm interested in has been really therapeutic. That's one of the things that I would probably attribute to a kind of postmenopausal liberation, being able to go, "Fuck it. This is who I am. I'm putting it on the page. And if you don't like it, you don't have to read it."

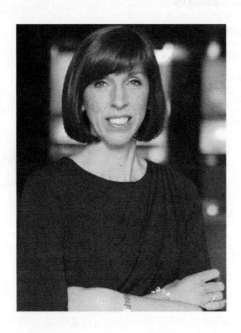

Louise Newson

Menopause specialist

"I love my family. But at the time you've got this demon in your brain telling you that what you're doing needs to be done. You don't care about anything else."

Dr Louise Newson is passionate about improving education about the perimenopause and menopause and also improving awareness of safe prescribing of HRT among healthcare professionals. She is author of *Menopause: All You Need to Know in One Concise Manual.* Louise started experiencing menopause symptoms in her mid-forties while she was in the early days of setting up her private menopause clinic and her Menopause Doctor website. But back then even she didn't register the symptoms.

~

It was something my daughter said that made me realise I must be perimenopausal – which is a bit embarrassing really. I'm a GP, not a gynaecologist, and I set up a menopause clinic around three years ago on my own. It was triggered by really wanting to help some of my menopausal friends who kept being given antidepressants, which I knew was wrong. Suddenly, I was seeing all these women coming into the clinic with dreadful symptoms, so I decided I wanted to write a website, menopausedoctor.co.uk, because I was disappointed with all the incorrect information that was out there for women, and for men. Writing content for the site was a huge job and, because I was doing the clinic as well, I was very tired.

But I was also more tired than usual. I kept thinking to myself, I feel drugged, I can't stay awake. I feel like I'm pregnant again, but I know I'm not.

I was really tired, really irritable, shouting all the time, tearful, emotionally labile. My memory was dreadful. I kept forgetting to take my daughter to her choir practice. I kept forgetting swimming kit for them to take to school. I kept even forgetting names for drugs I usually prescribe for my patients. And I kept looking at my examination couch and thinking, I need to go to sleep, I'm so tired. I had back-to-back migraines. I usually practise yoga regularly, but my muscles and joints were very stiff and sore. I felt very apathetic. I wanted to set up the clinic, but I just was too tired.

This went on for about four months and then one evening my daughter was on her phone. I said, "Come on, Sophie, you've got to go to bed." I was shouting and shouting. She said, "Mum, you're just so cross all the time. I think you need your period because some of my friends get really cross a bit like you before their periods."

Then I suddenly thought, Oh gosh, yes. I haven't had a period for about four months. I was having all these symptoms I just mentioned and I was also experiencing night sweats. I would often be waking up in the night so damp I felt like I had wet myself, and I'm not a sweaty person. It was absolutely vile.

As a doctor you always think there's something wrong with you, so I had thought I had lymphoma, which is a kind of cancer, and people with lymphoma often have night sweats. I kept thinking, I can't go to the doctors. I'm tired, I've got these other symptoms, I don't want to have a blood test because it might pick up something awful – and I'm too busy to be ill.

I didn't even piece it together. Meanwhile, the ironic thing is that I was writing all the time for my menopause website about all these symptoms that I actually had and how they start in women's forties and I was in my forties. I was forty-five at the time. I never used to track my periods. I never wrote them down. You just don't think about yourself, do you?

Age is really a number and I don't think of myself as a middle-aged woman. I didn't imagine I was there yet. But then I have also thought about all the younger women who might be going through it. One in a hundred women under the age of forty have an early menopause, so actually when you're in your thirties and experience these symptoms, it's no surprise that many women don't understand what is happening to them.

The symptoms, for me, were quite scary. I've been with my husband since I was eighteen, and suddenly I hated him. Even his breathing was annoying me. I could not stand anything about him. We went down to London with our family one weekend and I just remember there was something very trivial he said that really irritated me and I can't remember what it was but I started shouting and the children said, "Mummy, please don't shout like this, otherwise you'll get a divorce."

I said, "I don't care. Look at him. He is so annoying!"

My now seventeen-year-old daughter was talking about this the other day, and she said, "I was thinking if they get divorced you normally have to go with the mother and I don't want to go with Mum and I don't know what to do. It's really hard. But then I was worried as Daddy can't cook!"

She had all these thoughts. It's awful. I look back and I think, I didn't want to be divorced. What would I have done? I love my family. But at the time you've got this demon in your brain telling you that what you're doing needs to be done. You don't care about anything else.

I see so many women in my clinic who have separated from their partners and so many women who live with their partners and don't love them in the same way they used to and their relationships have changed. I can see how it happens. My ability to function as a working woman was affected. It was so hard. I would have definitely given up my job if I hadn't been able to get help.

I did a lot of work with West Midlands Police. We did a survey and nearly 80 per cent of women had had symptoms affecting their ability to work and about 25 per cent had given up their work, which is shocking. We know there are more men on senior boards than women and I'm sure much of it is a direct result of menopausal symptoms, which women aren't always recognising. Many women just think they're stressed at work or they can't cope with their lives, without understanding about the perimenopause and menopause.

Then, when I realised I had these symptoms, I thought, Well, what on earth am I going to do? My local GPs are really anti-HRT for the wrong reasons. Then I decided I would go and see Nick Panay, who is a consultant in London, because I know him very well. I phoned his clinic, and – like me – he has a six-month waiting list. This was in June and his secretary said, "Oh his next appointment is 24th December."

I said, "Oh, for goodness' sake, do you not know who I am? It's ridiculous, I can't wait that long." I was really cross and rude.

I was basically completely perimenopausal. I slammed down the phone and emailed Nick and said, "I'm really sorry, I need some HRT." He agreed to do a phone consultation with me in the next few days. But then I even forgot to phone him at the right time. Ten minutes before the appointment, I was with my daughter, out in London, and I said to her, "Look, in ten minutes I've got to make this really important phone call."

She said, "Yeah, whatever, fine."

The appointment was scheduled for nine. At ten past nine, Nick calls me and says, "Louise, weren't you going to phone me?" I said, "Oh no, I completely forgot." That's how badly my brain was not functioning. Then he advised me and I started HRT. I changed my dose and added in testosterone, and it wasn't until after I'd been taking it for six months, when I felt so much better, that I realised I actually must have been experiencing symptoms for about five or six years.

It's quite shocking. My own experience has driven me to work even harder because I think it's inexcusable that women are suffering, trying to live without hormones that are integral to their lives.

I've never worked this hard. I'm working so hard at the moment, but I can still cope with it because my brain is clear, my energy is really good, my sleep pattern is excellent. And that's because I take HRT. I could not function properly without it.

It's not like getting a nice haircut – where you want the best hairdresser and your hair to look good – this is our health and our future health.

A lot of women are scared of HRT for the wrong reasons. Many women think, I don't have many symptoms, maybe it doesn't matter. But actually it's a hormone replacement and we'll have low hormones for the rest of our lives, which we're not designed to have. We used to die not long after our menopause in the Victorian times. If I told you that you had iron deficiency, you would take iron. If it was a Vitamin D deficiency causing your symptoms, you would take Vitamin D. Women have a female hormone deficiency when they've gone through the menopause and because of the hormone deficiency there's an increased risk of heart disease, diabetes, depression, osteoporosis. The evidence is that the earlier you take HRT the better, because you get a really rapid reduction in bone density when your periods start changing.

I tweaked my HRT to make it work for me. Taking the right type and dose of HRT has enabled me to carry on having a healthy life – whereas I know I would have probably given up yoga, wouldn't have eaten so healthily and so on. My sleep was very interrupted even when I wasn't having the night sweats and we know that people who don't get enough sleep have a higher risk of all sorts of conditions including cancer, depression, heart disease, obesity.

I feel fine now. I'm not aware of any symptoms and if I wasn't doing all this menopause work, I wouldn't even think about my hormones.

I'm fifty years old now. The youngest patient I've seen at my clinic is just eighteen and she had a cancer at fourteen, which led to her having an early menopause. But then my oldest patient is ninety-four. The menopause affects us for so long. For most women it's a third of their lives, but for some women it's more than half, and we receive a large amount of input from doctors and healthcare professionals when we're pregnant for nine months or when we're needing contraception for maybe twenty to thirty years, but actually it's really important to get the menopause right – not just with HRT but with the right lifestyle advice.

People talk about the menopause as a taboo. But I think it's less of a taboo than a misunderstanding. I really want to rebrand the menopause because I think "menopause" is a horrible word. We shouldn't be making people feel bad. We should be talking about it as a female hormone deficiency that lasts long term. If women have an underactive thyroid gland then we diagnose hypothyroidism and we replace the thyroid hormone forever.

We should be more open talking about all the symptoms – the psychological symptoms, the lack of libido, the vaginal dryness. The majority of women have vaginal dryness if they're not on HRT, about 80 per cent, whereas only 8 per cent get treatment. I see women who can't sit down, who can't wear underclothes, who can't go cycling or swimming because they've got such severe symptoms – yet they're not receiving treatment. It's about improving knowledge and education.

I also see a lot of women in my clinic who have severe and crippling anxiety, and low mood as well. I see many women who have considered suicide. We know that the average age of menopause in the UK is fifty-one and we also know that the average age of suicides in the UK is early fifties. I've heard harrowing stories about women who have actually taken their lives when they've been menopausal and have been unable to receive the right help and treatment. I know it's related to hormones, because when you give these women HRT then often their moods really improve. But if people don't join the dots, they don't realise. Of course, they're not going to think it's related to hormones because they've not grown up thinking about it.

Most of the women who come to my clinic come because they aren't getting the right help from their own healthcare professionals – and my clinic is private because there aren't enough resources for NHS menopause care. I can't get a job in the NHS as a menopause specialist, which is outrageous.

The majority of women I see in my clinic end up taking HRT, because for the majority of women the health benefits of HRT outweigh any risks. The group of women who shouldn't take HRT first line [as a standard first treatment] are women who have had an oestrogen-receptive cancer in the past, but some women even choose to take HRT then as their menopausal symptoms are having such adverse effects on the quality of their lives. There are very few women who can't take HRT and, because of the health benefits HRT affords, the majority of women should consider taking it.

I prescribe body-identical hormones. Compounded bioidentical hormones are available in a lot of private clinics. They're not licensed, they're not regulated. They shouldn't be given at all. There is no evidence that they are better. We prescribe body-identical hormones, which are regulated products with evidence behind them. Some people you talk to, I'm sure, will be taking these compounded bioidentical hormones, and these women often do feel better because they do contain some oestrogen. But they are not safe and are not recommended.

I don't really have a problem with being older. Many of my friends would say, when I started taking HRT, "Doesn't that make you feel like you are getting old?" No. They said, "Oh, but you can't have children." And I said, "Well, I've been sterilised, I've had three children. I don't want to have one at forty-five. I had one at forty, that felt old enough."

> It's nothing to be ashamed of. It's a natural process.

Even some doctors say, "Gosh, you're really open about your own experience." Well, why wouldn't I be? It's nothing to be ashamed of. It's a natural process. I'm not here saying that everyone has to take HRT. Not everyone wants to, like not everyone wants to do yoga. It's about choice, and a lot of women aren't being given the choice, which is totally wrong.

It's interesting that my children, because all I do is talk about the menopause, are very educated about it. They're now recognising the menopause in many of their friends' mothers. My daughter, the other day, heard that her friend's mum was really moody and irritable. She was really struggling and had started to take some sage tablets. My daughter said to me, "I told her. She needs to take some HRT."

I think it's really great that my daughters are aware of the menopause because it's going to happen to them. It makes a big difference knowing about it. Because it can have a massive impact on their lives and future health. If you're dealing with it alone, the menopause can be very hard.

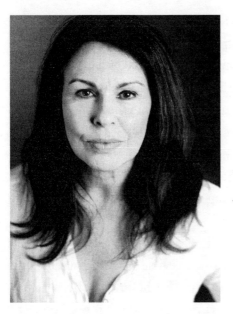

Julie Graham

Actor

"I can only describe it as having a tantrum. It's like a furnace within. A heat furnace that starts in your belly and you basically just have a big motherfucking tantrum."

Julie Graham, 55, wrote and starred in the online menopausal comedy-drama, *Dun Breedin*. She is best known for her roles in *At Home with the Braithwaites*, *Benidorm* and *Doc Martin*. In her late forties a close friend died suddenly, and soon after Joseph Bennett – her husband, and father of her two daughters – took his own life. In the years that followed she wasn't sure what was grief and anxiety over these losses, and what was perimenopause.

~

I'd had symptoms for a while and not really recognised them. What I always find strange about the menopause is that when you're coming up to puberty you have a conversation with your mum – whoever is the significant female in your life will talk with you – about periods and how at some point you're going to bleed and all the hideousness that can come with that. You're prepared for it in a way. I'm talking about the majority here – I know there are people who are not prepared. But with the menopause, we never really have that conversation with anyone. Well, I certainly hadn't – apart from one friend who had gone through it.

When you get to forty-nine or fifty, you're living your life and not expecting it – so when these things start happening to you, you just assume it's something else. I'd had a really tough couple of years . . . and I thought I was maybe having a delayed reaction to the death of a close friend and the death by suicide of my husband, Joseph, and having to move house, and all of the things that go with that. I thought I needed a bit of therapy, because I started having this terrible anxiety which I'd never had in my life before. I'm not a person who suffers from anxiety. I've been very lucky in that respect. But I had this low-level anxiety. I was worrying about things that I never worried about before and then not being able to sleep and thinking it was the anxiety keeping me awake. I thought it was attached to grief.

I thought it was post-traumatic stress. The weird thing was, at that point, I was doing a job I really loved and I was with people I really loved and I'd met a new partner. So, ostensibly on the outside, everything seemed to be going great and I should have been over the moon and happy about things and moving on and all that sort of stuff. But I would just wake up with this feeling of dread.

I never properly got the hot flushes. Well, I did to a certain extent in that I was much hotter than I usually am. But I would just get this uncontrollable rage. Oh my God, it would be disproportionate to the thing that had made me angry. The first time I had it I'd dropped something on my foot and it hurt and instead of going, "Ah that fucking hurt," I just went into this rage. It tipped me over.

My children were in the house and they looked at me and they were like, "What is going on?" These were other incidents. Just bursting into tears for no reason. Then my friend Hazel came to stay with me and she was the one who had really suffered during the menopause – and I'd seen her suffering and I knew she was on HRT, but the penny hadn't dropped. Because I was only fifty by that point.

It was Hazel who said to me, "Have your periods stopped?" I said, "Actually, yes, I haven't had a period for about three months. When I went to my GP, he told me don't come and see me until you've stopped your periods for a year." And Hazel said, "Go see another bloody doctor!"

So I went down to the surgery. I had an appointment with him, but it was only when I went into the surgery that I realised it was him again. That was the other thing: I couldn't remember anybody's name. I had fog brain. I went up to the receptionists. They said, "What are you here for?" I said, "I'm here to talk about the menopause." They said, "Oh, you don't want to see him. Cancel the appointment. And go and see Dr Howarth – she's brilliant."

So I did, and I described all the symptoms. She said, "When was your last period?"

I said, "Three months ago, but I've been told you need to have stopped your period for a year."

She said, "That's absolute rubbish." She'd just done a course at the Chelsea and Westminster menopause clinic, which was a happy accident. She then asked, "When do you want to start taking HRT?"

I said, "Don't you need to do tests?"

"Absolutely not," she said. "You've just described classic menopausal symptoms and you shouldn't be suffering."

Then I had this amazing conversation with her where she said she thought that women – and this was the new way of thinking – should start taking HRT before they hit the menopause. They should start taking it when they're perimenopausal, so they don't have to go through any of these awful symptoms.

I started taking it because I had got to the point where I thought my relationship with my new partner was going to break up. He was thirty-five at the time and he must have been thinking, What have I got myself into? I met this wonderful woman and she was lovely and funny and sexy and now she's turned into this mad bitch.

He never said anything like that, but I could feel it. I could feel his confusion. But when you're in the middle of it, you can't sit down and have a rational conversation about it. I was in denial a bit.

Then, when I started taking HRT, within about two weeks I felt normal again.

There is a lot of grief mixed up with the menopause for me. Not just my husband, but also my best friend – my closest friend in the whole world – died very suddenly. I spoke to her one morning – and she was dead by the afternoon. She had a catastrophic asthma attack which then led to heart failure; it happened when she was with her young daughter in a café. And I'd literally spoken to her about two hours before.

It's just such a terrible shock – and if grief impacts you mentally of course it's going to impact you physically as well. I remember the days and weeks after it happened, I was running on huge amounts of adrenaline to keep me going. We organised the funeral and all that sort of stuff. Then you go back to normal life, and I had a terrible crash. My body gave up because, as I say, I was running on adrenaline and grief.

Looking back, I have no idea how I managed, because I was forty-eight when that happened. Then, six months later, my husband, the father of my children, took his own life. And we were in the middle of moving house, then our dog died, then my cousin died of cancer very, very quickly and I know this sounds ridiculous but our campervan burned down and it was like the last straw. I was thinking, Are you fucking kidding me? I was ranting and raving at the universe, going, "Fuck off, stop doing this to me!"

I have no idea if I was suffering perimenopausal symptoms because it was hard to tell things apart. It wasn't until I met somebody and I was in a good place and I'd moved house and I was quite settled that it became clear I was just a basket case.

But I have to say, within two weeks of taking HRT, I felt normal again.

The sleep deprivation was driving me insane as well because I've always been a person who needs to sleep and I was operating on very little. Then that would lead into the rage and the anger. So it was like a kind of vicious cycle.

But then, after about a year of taking HRT, I noticed the symptoms started coming back. By then I was able to recognise it. So I went back to my GP, who said, "I think we need to up the dose." She did that and within a week of taking the new dose, I felt back to normal.

Now I know the difference between the symptoms of menopause and normal everyday somebody-at-the-post-office pissing me off. Now they just piss me off. Whereas before I wanted to kill them. Now, I get a normal level of annoyance, rather than murderous intent.

It's like being a toddler and having no control over your faculties because you've got no way to express yourself. You're taught from a very young age, especially girls and women, that you should be well-behaved and polite, so it goes against your innate social skills to be uncontrollable and incandescent with rage. I can only describe it as having a tantrum. It's like a furnace within. A heat furnace that starts in your belly and you basically just have a big motherfucking tantrum.

It's really upsetting afterwards. It's like when toddlers have a tantrum and they sleep for about an hour, because they're so exhausted. That's what happens. I'm so exhausted by the rage and it also triggers a huge emotional reaction because you feel quite embarrassed – at the way you've behaved and reacted.

I don't think that rage is ever useful. There's a difference between rage and anger, and I think uncontrollable rage is just very, very detrimental, not only to other people but to your own health and mental health. Whereas anger is a different thing. Righteous anger, that's part of getting older, of having the confidence to express it and point out injustice. Also, you know yourself, that when you see someone losing control, whether that's a man or a woman, the minute they do that, when they're ranting and raving, you lose respect and stop listening. So it doesn't really get you anywhere.

I feel absolutely no sense of loss over my fertility. Maybe that's because I had children late. My first child was born when I was thirty-nine and my second child when I was nearly forty-one, so I guess I felt lucky. I didn't have any sense of, "Oh God, that's the end of my fertility."

I don't miss my periods at all. To be perfectly honest, I've been lucky in that even when I had periods they were very manageable. Still, I'm so pleased they're gone. Perhaps that's another reason the menopause was such a shock to my system – in that I didn't really have PMT. I never got bad cramps or anything. I never suffered in the way I've seen a lot of my friends suffer.

When my periods were getting erratic and stopping, because I was in the middle of all that loss and grief and turmoil, I wasn't keeping track of them and sometimes I wouldn't know when it was one month to the next. So I'd have a period and I'd ask myself, "Maybe I didn't have a period last month?" I probably did think I was perimenopausal but I assumed that was just about periods. I didn't realise you got symptoms. That's how ignorant I was about it.

I don't want my daughters growing up in the same way that I grew up, not knowing about the menopause. I want them to be able to have a conversation about it, to recognise when it's happening to them and do something about it. Hopefully the medical professionals will have moved on by then, too.

But even though I was going through the menopause in my life and so were my friends, the one place I didn't see it was on television.

The only time a menopausal woman was on television was when she was the butt of a joke. She was usually in her sixties and a little bit overweight, angry and having a hot flush – someone to be ridiculed. It was always from the male gaze. I got fed up not seeing myself on screen and I got fed up with the parts drying up because I was over fifty. I thought, Why not kill two birds with one stone? I'll create great parts for older women and have a conversation about the menopause.

It seemed like a no-brainer to me and I started writing *Dun Breedin*.

It's a television comedy about a group of friends all going through different stages and symptoms of the menopause. During the Covid-19 lockdown we decided to go ahead and film a kind of pilot version to go online.

I wanted to portray the experience that our generation is having and not my mother's generation, because my mother's generation is the one that was heavily medicated through the menopause. My aunt Isabel, my aunt May, all of them would have cabinets full of pills. They would go to their GPs and the GP would give them Valium and sleeping pills and they would be medicated through it. But it was the menopause they were going through: they weren't depressed; they weren't anxious. They were having all these symptoms and the GPs would say, "Have a tablet, mother's little helper." Or they would drink their way through it because they didn't know what was happening to them because nobody talked about it.

Another reason I wanted to write *Dun Breedin* was to say, "It's not all over." Once we stop bleeding, once we stop having children, once we go through the menopause, it's not over. In fact, it can be a very empowering time. It can be a very creative time and a very sexy time. So many women talk about having sex without worrying about getting pregnant. Or simply discovering their sexuality again. It's not all negative. There are quite positive things.

I'm in a relatively new relationship with a younger man, so that has had a positive impact on my libido. In a lot of relationships people are together for an age and men's libido drops as well, and there's a dip to do with a long-term relationship. But the loss of libido can absolutely be down to a physical symptom of the imbalance of hormones. And what's also not talked about is that it can also partly be the psychological impact of weight gain – your waist thickening, putting on weight for no reason. That can really affect your self-confidence, and therefore your libido. All these things are connected yet we treat them completely separately as symptomatic rather than in a holistic way. I think that's how the menopause needs to be treated: holistically.

> We are very much an ignored majority.

Also, with *Dun Breedin*, I wanted to write about real women and real relationships. I wanted to write about people putting on weight and weeing themselves because their pelvic floor is a bit off, things I never see reflected on screen. We are very much an ignored majority.

I don't want people to laugh at me, I want them to laugh with me. I felt if I was going to make people laugh about menopause then it was going to be my joke. Comedy can open up the conversation in a more gentle way because people feel they can have a laugh about it rather than taking it as a very serious subject, which of course it is. Because society has taught us to feel a certain amount of embarrassment or shame about it, there's a whole conspiracy of silence around the menopause that I find very disturbing.

For me, the menopause has been the beginning of something. I'd always wanted to write and never got round to it. Because of life events – and, to be honest, any excuse under the sun – I'd not written before. But actually this has hopefully given me a whole new career, which I don't think I would have done before I went through the menopause. So, you know, it's given something back to me.

It's important we have this conversation because it's not just women who go through the menopause – their partners go through it with them. Their husbands, their wives – all go through it with them. Their children go through it with them. At least if you can have a conversation, there can be more empathy within the relationship. I remember having one conversation with Davy, afterwards. I addressed it. I remember him saying he'd felt sorry for me. And initially I had a terrible gut reaction to that. But he didn't mean he pitied me – he meant he felt for me, going through something he had no control over. And so at least when I addressed it, we could talk about it.

Both my daughters are teenagers, so they're going through their own hormonal hells sometimes. It's been very loud in our house at times. Of course, we have very open conversations about it. We have a laugh. They say, "For fuck's sake – have I got this to look forward to?" I'm like, "Yeah, but knowledge is power. If you know what's coming at least you can deal with it." Also if they see a success story – if they see their mother dealing with it in a good way and coming out the other side and still being vital and creative and alive – then they won't be fearful of it. Because there's nothing to be scared of.

It has made me reflect on my relationship with my own mother. Unfortunately she died when I was eighteen, of cancer. For about a year and a half before she died, we had a very adversarial relationship. And I realise now that she was probably going through the menopause and I was going through being an absolute twat teenager. Of course, hindsight is a great thing and I wish that I'd known.

Maybe it wouldn't have made a blind bit of difference, but the point is I just thought she was being unreasonable and she thought I was a teenage nightmare. Which I was – but I didn't realise she was going through anything of her own. I thought she was over-reacting to everything.

The only time I ever heard menopause mentioned was when my aunties would say, "Oh, she's going through the change." In my teenage brain I didn't even think to wonder what "the change" was. I just knew it was something secretive and probably not very nice because it was always talked about in either hushed tones or a negative context.

The other thing that I've done in this phase is be a bit more selfish. I've thought, You know what, I've raised two daughters, done my bit, and I can have a little bit more time to myself. I think a lot of women have the touch of the martyr to them – and it's a little bit *poor me*. I actually just think, shut up and go and have a fucking massage. One of the things I do is take time for myself, go for a walk on my own to the beach, have a pamper day, ring friends up and say, "Let's have a spa day." I do things for me. If I've got a day off that's what I'll do rather than sorting out my bills. I'm not just talking about women, it's for men too. It's just that I think women tend to put too much on themselves. When someone asked me recently what I would keep from this time of Covid, I said, "I will keep socially distancing myself from wankers." We've got to take that attitude a little bit for ourselves.

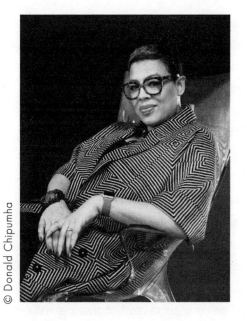

India Gary-Martin

Leadership coach

"I lose my shit. Things frustrate me and I get really mad. Order is important to me."

India Gary-Martin, 50, is a globally recognised leadership expert and coach with a clientele of Fortune 500 and C-Suite executives from around the world. She has three children and recently moved back to her home country of the United States, where she found herself going through grief, lockdown and perimenopause.

~

I do have rage. I did a lot of stressful things you're not supposed to do all together within months. I moved not just house, but country, back from the UK to the United States. Also my brother died. So I'm not sure whether my behaviour has been as a result of response to stressors, or if it was the perimenopause or menopause.

I get rage that goes go from zero to sixty in milliseconds. My labile mood swings are outrageous. My triggers are really light. I'll get triggered and then afterwards. I'm like, "Who was that person? How did that happen?" I can't control it.

It could just be my kids making too much noise. My office in my house is downstairs in the basement, and so our living area is right above me, and they'll be running around with dogs while I'm trying to have meetings and record. They're eleven and fourteen, they're not babies, and they are literally like wild horses running through my house.

I lose my shit. Things frustrate me and I get really mad. Order is important to me: I don't like a whole bunch of madness and wildness in our house. My husband and I both feel like everything has its place and should be put back there. So I find that when those things don't happen it's acute for me. I get really annoyed when things aren't where they're supposed to be or when kids leave things lying around – which they do because they are kids.

I've said really rude things to my kids. It's actually horrible, because I think about how that would feel if my mum said those things to me. My mum didn't say crazy things to me. She managed it. I'm trying to find the tools to manage it like her. The most she would say was, "You can cut that shit out." That wasn't so bad; in my case, a plethora of four-letter words seems to have become my specialty.

I know that it's beyond my control because I know this is not my idea of what I would do. That's not what I'd want to feel. I wouldn't want anybody saying that to me in that tone, in that way, but it's out of my control – because it's my hormones. And I feel sad afterwards. I feel badly because I don't want to be saying that to them. I don't want that to be their experience: a crazy mum who is effing and blinding all the time.

I'm sure I'm perimenopausal, but I still have completely regular cycles every single month like clockwork. I've noticed they're a little bit heavier and the cramps are like I am thirteen again. What the hell? I think it's because I have fibroids. I've had them removed twice and if I were to have them removed again that would be my third time – though I'm not going to do it. I'll have to have the full hysterectomy now. I'm thinking, I know I'm going to go into menopause anyway so it doesn't really matter if I go directly there because I've had the hysterectomy . . .

> I'm so excited about becoming an elder – though I'm not there yet.

I had night sweats really early, in my early forties, but not now – those were sweats where I'd wake up and my entire bed would be drenched and I'd have changed my clothes and put a towel down because I would be wet through, literally drenched in my clothes. I'd have to get up and change, and then put a towel on my bed; I couldn't be changing the sheets because my husband was sleeping. But that stopped, I haven't had it for a while, and I don't have any flushes.

I've had adult acne. When my period comes I'm getting full-blown pimples. I'm like, "That is not okay. What am I . . . a teenager?"

I'm able to control my rage at work. I can manage people in work situations, but I cannot manage random people in general. I've had this anger at people not wearing Covid-19 masks. If I go somewhere and somebody doesn't have a mask on and it doesn't seem like there's a legitimate reason I am that person who will go into that rage thing. I get really angry. I go off into talks about my health and how they're impacting my health. I have gone full-blown effing and blinding with no filters.

That's been one of the struggles: moving to the US in such crazy times, arriving here in the time of Trump and Covid-19, the foolishness going on in this country . . . What's wrong with these people?

I've talked a lot about the menopause with my friends both sides of the Atlantic. I have a very open mother, so she's been my barometer for talking about things. She's more open than most people in general. She talks about anything. She asked me how my sex life was when I first got married. No thanks, Mom.

I'm the same with my kids – very open. And they hate it, really hate it. My teenage daughter is going through the same hormonal changes at the other end, coming into it. We have some real clashes, she and I, because, if her cycle is coming, she is an absolute cow, and I'm just hoping I don't get one of my mood swings because then I may be one second away from doing my jujitsu body slams.

I'm so excited about becoming an elder – though I'm not there yet. I'm excited about that transition because I'm already aware of the wisdom, the things that I know now that I wish I'd known when I was younger.

I know that I'm getting older. I'm not as cute as I once was to people, not as physically attractive perhaps in some ways, but I don't care – because I'm having such a good time. That whole being able to walk through life and not give a toss is so wonderful. It is so freeing. I have so much freedom because I care not what anybody thinks about any of it. Getting older, for me, I see as liberation from what, when you're younger, you think you have to conform to.

Partly the future seems so promising because of my mum and my grandma. My grandma was a twin and she died two years ago at ninety-seven. Her twin is ninety-nine and will be a hundred in February 2021, but is still as lucid as anything. She thinks George Clooney is cute, and she's saying things like, "Ooh, I can have a little bit of that." She's hilarious. So I see some kind of freedom in the fact that I might have the trajectory of the women in my family. If I live that long, I could only be halfway through right now. I could have a whole other half to go.

I think this could be fun, as long as your body doesn't fail you. My great aunt, who I call my grandma too, her body hasn't failed her, and she's very well loved and taken care of and she lives in our family home. She's not in a nursing home, so she's having a good time.

I am very much part of my family culture. We live very multi-generationally. The plan is for my parents to move in with me. We do have a real pecking order of where we fall in the family in terms of age and a whole bunch of other things. It's really a very distinct culture and it's driven by Creole culture. My mum's family is from New Orleans.

I'm so excited that my parents are going to move in with me; that my mother will be here cooking and my dad will be here smoking a cigar. Let me be clear, they do get on my nerves, but it's just going to be such a wonderful thing for my kids to be able to have that multi-generational impact and wisdom, and that support and attention and love all the time. For me working, too, it's useful to have my mum around.

My mum does work, by the way. The woman will not stop working. She consults and she is on boards and she's still quite active. She'll never stop. She's like Ruth Bader Ginsburg, the Supreme Court Justice, RIP. She'll just keep doing whatever – influencing is what she calls it.

Attitudes towards older or menopausal women in business are actually pretty horrible. The idea that we do have a shelf life exists today, and once a woman hits a certain age people start to be dismissive. But, in some ways, I'm really lucky, because people don't know what age I am unless I tell them. It's the same for my mum; people fully believe she should still be working and she's seventy-four, but she looks like she's fifty. I think I've slid by some of that, because I still look much younger than I am. But it is hard and I think that women do suffer that "shelf life" idea terribly.

I'm hoping that in the US, with the real focus there now on race – the UK has a much longer way to go with these conversations – if we can get that right, which is the hardest thing, then it helps all of the other diversity pillars including gender. The civil rights movement gave way to the birth of the feminist movement in the US, because it created all the civil liberties that the feminist groups needed.

Here in the US there are some pretty horrific statistics about health inequity for ethnic communities, and that impacts on experience of the menopause, especially given that there's not universal health care. You get women who are really suffering through menopause, but who are unable to access any of the support that you would need to help. This typically happens in lower-income Black and Latino communities and Indigenous communities – they don't have access to any of the tools or resources and also because menopause isn't something that is part of a mainstream conversation.

I think we need to recognise menopause as a condition, a natural part of what women go through; just like girls coming into their hormones and periods should be recognised as a condition too.

I am the US co-chair of Women of the World (WOW), and we've had lots of sessions on menopause. I think there's a real opportunity for a movement here, just like period poverty became a real movement out of WOW, a massive movement. I'm thinking, *How do we make menopause a bigger one?*

FOG

(noun)

c.f. Brain fog. An inability to think clearly, focus or remember anything at all, including whether you have put the keys in the fridge.

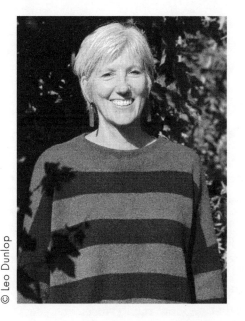

Pippa Marriott

Teacher

*"It was like I'd lost
my nerve."*

Pippa Marriott, 58, is a former senior teacher who found the perfect storm of menopausal insomnia, anxiety and brain fog made her question her abilities at work. A mounting sense of low-level panic contributed to her decision to quit her job and take early retirement.

~

I was teaching drama at a large girls' school. I mention that it was a girls' school because that came to feel important later on as I realised that actually I had a responsibility to those students in terms of my own responses to ageing. Rather than hiding menopause and ageing, I should be honest and open about it.

My main sense around it was of embarrassment, and also a deeper emotion than simply embarrassment: I felt shame. I was on the senior leadership team at the school and I remember people talking

43

about this idea that our staff room was full of menopausal women, and me, shamefully, not really challenging that.

I laughed it off in the same way that when you're a child and bullying is going on you share the "joke" because you think: If I don't join in, I'm potentially the victim in this. What I didn't do was challenge it. There was a real element of not wanting to be associated with the menopause and the whole baggage of stuff attached to that comment, the careless mockery and disrespect that went with it.

Also, with my colleagues who were struggling with sweats and hot flushes, I was sympathetic to them but also, I'm ashamed to say, there was initially an unsisterly part of me that just didn't want to know. Almost like I didn't want to catch it off them! I didn't want to step over that line or join that club. I'm fessing up to the fact that, pre-menopause, I wanted to distance myself from that step into menopause.

Later, I experienced hot flushes, but not, thankfully, drenching sweats. My sleep patterns, however, were hugely affected. I soon identified as a menopause symptom this kind of shot of cortisol which I'd get at various points in the night. I'd be waking up – often eight times a night – and lying there completely wide awake. Of course, when you're in a high-pressured job your brain is immediately on, thinking about all these things: "I must send that email. What am I going to do with the Year 8s? I've got to have a difficult conversation with so-and-so." You eventually get back to sleep, but then you're awake again thinking, Oh, it's five o'clock and I've got to be up at six o'clock. I must get a bit more sleep.

The effects of sleep deprivation started leaking into my day – leaking in in terms of someone coming to my office for a meeting and me saying, "Great, lovely to see you, sit down," while thinking, I have no memory of booking this meeting!

Teaching is an exposed job. You're very much on show every day, not just with students, but also with staff.

A part of my role involved meeting and greeting parents and showing people around the school and so on, as well as dealing with hundreds of students. Mostly with the students I didn't have a problem remembering their names but once my brain was alerted to a sense of doubt, that I couldn't quite trust myself to remember things, I'd be looking at someone and thinking, God, I think it's Vicky . . . But is it Vicky or is it Vanessa? It's probably not the one I'm thinking it is . . .

There was a quiet panic that set in because I couldn't trust my brain in the ways that I always had previously. And as a teacher when there are so many interactions in the day, you are utterly reliant on firing on all cylinders and holding those forty-eight things in your brain that need to be there. So, once I knew that my brain could forget I'd booked a meeting with someone, I lost confidence in my ability to retain all the masses of information I should have had at my fingertips. There weren't any major or even minor fuck-ups, but I had this creeping fear that I couldn't trust my brain to retain things like I'd done so effortlessly in the past.

It was like I'd lost my nerve. I remember a particular time I took some sixth-formers into London. I'd done the risk assessment and so on, there was another teacher there, but I couldn't get rid of a feeling of panic. I was sweating, not because of a hot flush, but because of panic. On the Tube, I just kept counting the students. "Was that twelve? Fuck. Count them again." I thought, what has happened to me? I felt afterwards, something has changed. My innate confidence was rocked and that really unsettled me. I began to wonder whether this was actually some cognitive impairment.

I was about fifty-three and I remember going to the doctor and, as is quite often the case when you teach in a school, she was the mother of someone I had taught. I said to her, "I can't trust my faculties. What can I do about it? Is it early onset dementia?" She laughed it off, saying, "Well, you're in a stressful job, but you're great at what you do. There's not a problem."

I thought, Yeah, you don't get it. I'm not as great as I was. What's happened? Will that ever come back?

There were those shots of panic, and a deep, underlying anxiety and loss of confidence in myself. I was beginning to question, Can I do this?

Somewhere around this time, I bought Jenni Murray's *Is It Me, Or Is It Hot In Here?* for a friend's fiftieth, partly as a joke. I had a read of it first. Actually it was only reading the beginning, when she was describing someone at a meeting having brain freeze and forgetting the name of a really good friend of hers, that I thought, Oh God, so maybe I haven't got Alzheimer's. Maybe it's to do with menopause!

> And then my natural hair emerged and I felt really disloyal to this wonderful variegated grey that I had covered up for so long!

That was my first realisation that those slippages might not mean I was heading for dementia. I don't think I have ever been so relieved to have a menopausal symptom!

I later went back to my GP to talk to her about this and my sleep patterns, and she was very gung-ho about suggesting I go on HRT, in quite a refreshing way. That was a relief because HRT hadn't been something I ever thought I would take. Because of attitudes in my friendship groups and my route as an 1980s feminist, when we were all reading publications like *Our Bodies, Ourselves*, I just thought that won't be something I do, but I did, and it made a real difference.

At the same time, there was an issue going on with my hair. I don't dye my hair anymore, but then I was dyeing it to what had been its natural colour. After a few weeks, that badger stripe would reappear and I would jokingly refer to it as my line of shame! If I couldn't find time to dye my hair, I'd be walking with my head up in school, thinking, Don't look at the top of my head!

And then I thought, Here I am, a proud feminist woman spending a lot of time empowering my students about who they are and celebrating diversity and complexity, but actually I'm carrying this sense of shame about my natural hair colour! But how could I stop dyeing it? As a teacher your appearance is always noticed. You walk in the class and a student will say, "Oh, I like your earrings, Miss." They don't miss a trick, and they would certainly notice me going from auburn to full-on grey. Nonetheless, who was I kidding and what sort of role model was I being if I couldn't accept that I was in a natural ageing process?

At that point I thought, Right I'm going to have it cut really short, and then see what happens. And then my natural hair emerged and I felt really disloyal to this wonderful variegated grey that I had covered up for so long!

I still feel a bit embarrassed to admit that I take HRT. One of the reasons for this is that responses to menopause and ageing get polarised and put into boxes. On the one side you have the Wise Woman moving into spiritual enlightenment, all of that natural loveliness. And over towards the other side are lip fillers and Botox and interventionist stuff – all of which I absolutely wouldn't do, and I think I am quite judgemental of those who make those choices. But I feel HRT is on that side, so actually I am choosing an intervention. We all have to do the research and find our own way.

The reality is you can do a bit of both. You can do the Wise Woman and the HRT – and that's where I came to. I now take a pill every other day. HRT has really helped me. I couldn't have carried on with that fragmented sleep. It was literally doing my head in, and HRT ameliorated that.

At that time, when my symptoms were worst, my son was taking his GCSEs and we'd been planning to move to Devon, so it was a question of do we do it that summer, or does he take A levels first, and then we move. I felt I couldn't do two more years at senior teacher level, carrying that feeling that I've got to hold the whole sky up. I probably felt that 80 per cent of the time – this great weight of responsibility, underscored with a deep unease about my abilities.

So I made the decision to leave. I can't put all of that on to menopause, but it definitely shifted something, and made me re-evaluate things. I ended up working part-time at a school in Exeter and it was a joy not to have any of that added responsibility. After a while they started asking me to take on extra things and if I would go full-time and I thought, No. I'm not going to put myself in that position. I don't want to work in that way again.

I took early retirement at fifty-five years old. I'm now working freelance, as a writer and trainer. I also took a Master's at Exeter University, in creative writing, and alongside that I set up a creative writing group in Exeter prison, and I've been working more with community groups. I have refound my confidence.

I was always an activist and this phase has fired that up again and allowed more space for it. In that heat, almost, of the menopause, there's some kind of fire which brings about a reckoning, and things get swept away, and what are you left with? What are you doing next on your journey in your life?

Recently, with this whole fiasco over the Covid-19-era A level results, I found myself thinking, I want to be part of whatever the education revolution is that will come on the back of this, because this is symptomatic of an education system so fixated on assessment and grading that it places cohort statistics above individuals. In the past I have been very involved in looking at developments in education, so I felt something inside me go, "Yeah, actually, I would climb back on board to fight for an overhaul of our broken education system."

When we talk about diversity and inclusion, and deliver training on unconscious bias, we need to remember the women like us. We don't want to lose us from the workplace, these brilliant women in their fifties and their sixties with masses to give. I find myself wondering if it could have been different at work, at the school I was at. I feel partly culpable as I was in a position where I could have brought about some change in relation to that. It isn't good enough that senior leaders can sit and say, "Yeah, we've got a staff room full of menopausal women," and for me to be sitting around that table and not say, "Hang on a second, that's completely out of order." It's not right that I could sit shamefacedly thinking, Yeah I know exactly what you mean. That's not good enough. I could have been more honest and open myself.

I see menopause as a coming of age metaphorically and literally – it's a coming of ageing into your body and your mind and into yourself. As Mary Oliver says, "What is it you plan to do with your one wild and precious life?"

And, interestingly, lockdown has had some similar effects to menopause on our collective consciousness. Both seem to be saying, "Hang on a minute, time to take stock. What are you doing? Why are you doing this? Is this how you want to live?"

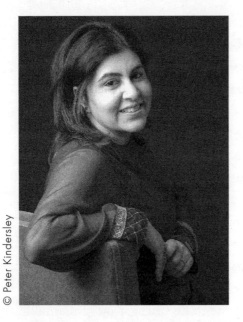

Sayeeda Warsi

Politician

*"I did find that Baroness
Warsi again. The fog
did clear."*

Baroness Sayeeda Warsi, 49, is a politician and member of the House
of Lords. She had ministerial roles in the Cameron–Clegg coalition.
In 2014 she resigned, citing her disagreement with the government's
policy on the Israel–Gaza conflict. She grew up in a family of Pakistani
Muslim immigrants living in West Yorkshire and had a first career as a
solicitor. She had one child during her first marriage and has brought
up a further four children with her current husband.

~

On my Instagram profile, I've posted the line, "Fighting injustice and
the menopause." That's because I do feel menopause is an injustice
we have to deal with as women. Many of us, when we get into our
forties, are firing on all cylinders in our careers. We are financially

better off than we have ever been. We are more in control of our lives and sure of ourselves than we have ever been. Then it hits. I felt like I was hit by a juggernaut. Suddenly I saw a side of myself that I didn't recognise. I thought, this isn't me. I was always the one that had tons of energy, was multitasking, could be thinking of ten things at the same time and now this had changed.

I probably started experiencing symptoms at the age of forty-six. Initially I thought it might just be a phase. *Maybe I'm a little bit tired,* I thought. *I just need to eat better.* Then, two summers ago, there was a big family wedding and, looking back at the photos and the video, I see I was constantly sat with a fan in my hand. It was a hot summer and it was a typical Asian wedding in that a lot of the outfits were very heavy and decorated and there was lots of jewellery and lots of makeup and I remember thinking, throughout the whole wedding, I am so *hot*.

The fan was a gift which had sat in my wardrobe for years and I never envisaged using it. But it was the only elegant way to cope with getting through the wedding that summer, which seemed to go on for weeks and weeks. During that time, I went to a private clinic. I had read up on something called bioidentical hormones, which are creams that you rub into your forearm and I felt like that may be slightly better than taking pills.

The cream seemed to work for a little while and then it stopped working. What I've realised over the past few years is that meno-pause comes in waves and you can do something, and you think it's worked and so carry on doing it, but it comes back again. I am currently going through a wave of symptoms, even though I am at my fittest and healthiest right now.

After I tried the bioidentical hormones, I started taking black cohosh, which is an herbal remedy, and then I started dealing with my health and fitness and eating better. Each approach seemed to work for a while. Each change I make initially works and holds back the symptoms, but then a few months later another wave of symptoms returns.

I found the hot sweats the most difficult, because I do a lot of face-to-face work. Oddly, this Covid-19 period has been easier because of Zoom calls, but I used to dread sitting in a meeting and thinking, God I'm going to burst into sweats, and this is really uncomfortable and it's probably visible on my face as well. Oddly, the more you worry about it, the worse it gets.

I do quite a lot of media and thankfully, so far, I haven't had any interviews when I had a hot flush, but I had lots and lots of meetings where I could feel myself heating up and feeling really uncomfortable.

But what I have struggled with in media interviews is sometimes simply losing the ability to construct sentences. Occasionally, I did a media interview and midway I lost words. I lost the ability to construct sentences. I would find myself stopping in the middle of an interview and thinking, I can't finish this because I can't put these words together. Only the year before, 2016/17, I had written a 120,000-word book in under twelve months, and yet here I was a year later struggling to construct simple sentences.

I found it helped to think things through carefully before I went on because I had lost confidence in my ability to construct things really quickly. I'm a lawyer. I've always been quick on my feet. I've always felt I was someone who could construct an argument coherently and quickly, but suddenly I felt I just couldn't do that.

For me it's been partly about embracing the fact that I can't be superwoman all the time. I have also had insomnia and what I started doing, rather than try to fight it, is just get up and work. So if I was awake at two a.m., I would think, I can either lie here and try to get back to sleep for hours, or I can actually get up and do some work and then when I'm tired go to sleep.

The only thing I can compare this to is the sleep deprivation that comes after having a baby. Again, there was this sense at that time that I must be superwoman. The symptoms were very similar: feeling really tired, wanting to do it all but not being able to do it, feeling like you were a bit of a failure because you couldn't do it all, trying to keep going in the same routine, when actually once you embrace sleeping when baby sleeps and waking when baby wakes it makes life a whole lot easier.

I also remember feeling really low. I probably had postnatal depression, though it was never diagnosed. I didn't take my low mood at that time seriously and neither did anyone else around me. When I did raise it, I was just told to pull myself together and get on with it. There was an expectation that as a woman I should have been naturally and instinctively maternal and that feeling low and unhappy was just me being awkward and that I shouldn't talk about it.

This time I thought to myself, I'm not prepared to let other people determine what is acceptable and what isn't acceptable, what's normal and what we can talk about. This time, from my own home, I'm going to start by having these conversations, initially at home and then more broadly, including now having a very public conversation, so this time it has been different.

The way I have dealt with facing this juggernaut of menopause was first of all deciding I needed to deal with it in my own immediate life, my home life. I took the decision to talk to my husband and talk to my kids about it, the boys and the girls. Our eldest is twenty-nine and our youngest is twenty-one, three boys and two girls. I told them to go away and read about it, which they did and then we discussed it. My husband did quite a lot of reading around the subject too.

What was important to me was to get to a point where we could talk about the menopause in a serious and informed way – because

I think even in the home, comments like, "Oh, Mum's just being menopausal . . . Mum's just being hormonal" meant that this really important and difficult phase could so easily be dismissed.

I felt we needed to move on from talking about it in a flippant way, whether it's in the home, or among friends, or in public.

What shocks me is how so many women must be going through this at any one point and yet it is such an under-discussed issue. I suppose we talk about it amongst our girlfriends, but even then, it's treated as a bit of a joke, rather than seriously discussing what we are going through and how we are dealing with it.

We need to talk about it in a serious way, saying that these are symptoms of a health condition that we need to understand because it has a real impact on the way in which we function on a day-to-day basis. And as women we just need to ask for help.

After I had my daughter, rather than ask for help, I tried to estab-lish some normality in my life and went back to work full-time when she was less than twelve weeks old. That was my way of dealing with it – to go back to work and get some routine in my life. It was probably a crazy way to do it, but in the end it kind of worked.

This time, with the menopause, I decided I was going to manage my work–life balance better and that more work was not going to be the answer. This time, I also had a lot of support around me; I am in a happy relationship and I took the decision to be upfront. I sought support and I let other people be part of the process rather than deal with it myself.

I have also focused on my lifestyle. I recently lost a lot of weight through diet and exercise. It's had a strong positive impact on my life. I feel lighter, I feel healthier, I feel stronger – all those things have got to be good for you. I lost it by weight training. I also changed the way I ate to a calorie-controlled and cleaner diet. It's just being more aware, drinking more water, being more active, making sure I get some steps in during the day, making exercise a core part of the week – prioritising me, not pushing it down the list. I made lots of small changes; there's no single magic pill.

For me, this was completely health-driven – I was pre-diabetic and had high blood pressure. Suddenly I had started to feel like I was quite a weak person. I wanted to feel stronger. And I felt the only way to feel stronger was weight training. I was struggling to carry heavy things. That was what hit me the most and what I wanted to change, to get the strength back. Because for me with strength came independence. I felt like losing strength was the first sign of dependency. Simple things, like my husband said I was grunting coming up the stairs – and all I was doing was taking the washing basket up! Now I feel that I can lift, walk with strength and have physical independence, which gives me choices. For me, it's about making sure in later life we don't lose those choices.

By the time we hit menopause, I feel women are better at knowing who we are and what we want. We should be able to handle things much better than any challenges we might have had in our twenties and thirties.

Many women by this time will be at the top of their careers, so there is an unfairness to menopause. Women do not want to be seen at that stage to be displaying the behaviour which menopausal symptoms bring about; for example, being uncomfortable in meetings, not being able to think clearly all the time, lack of energy, etc. Often these successful women are brushing the menopause under the carpet, because they think otherwise they will be supporting this attitude of "And this is why we don't promote women because this is how they behave . . . Oh God, she's having a day off." It can reignite that whole misogynistic approach to the "why women aren't equals in the workplace" debate.

It is unfair. I talked to my daughter, who is training to be a medic, and she is convinced that if men had the menopause we would have found all sorts of cures for it by now, all sorts of ways to deal with the symptoms. But, sadly, we still live in a world where any kind of emotional response in the workplace is considered bad and taboo and we have been conditioned over the years not to talk about our health, our feelings or our physical "shortcomings".

There are all sorts of taboos around women talking about menopause. I've spoken to older Asian women asking why they don't and a lot of them spoke about the fear of being infertile and therefore being "past it". Women, who had been homemakers and found their worth that way and through children, said that at a time their children were growing up and moving out and their body was telling them they could no longer produce children, they felt as if somehow their life had ended. It was tough to hear these conversations and yet we should be celebrating this moment. Celebrating the fact that the children have left home, the fact that we're now empty-nesters. And that finally we don't have to put up with a distraction of a period every month. I celebrated this phase in my life. My husband and I joke how we are reliving our youth.

We've been great empty-nesters. That's partly because, for us as a couple, and as individuals, the kids are a huge part of our lives, but they are not the only part of our life or even the biggest part. I've had friends who were really traumatised empty-nesters. I think menopause in women feeds into this because there is this sense of loss and end of an era. And the end of fertility I think is a big part of that.

Probably the most difficult thing for me is what I call head fog, the inability to think quickly and clearly. That ability was something I'd always taken for granted and I saw it as the basis for much of my success. I felt as an advocate, long before politics, that was who I am.

And because I felt I was losing that ability to articulate quickly and clearly and coherently and use language well, to use wit, all of that, I felt I was starting to lose a part of me that was integral to part of my personality.

I remember my daughter turning around to me one day and saying, "We need to find the Baroness Warsi again."

I asked her what she meant, because as a family we never use my title.

But what she was effectively saying was that we needed to find that publicly strong, independent, kick-ass, out-there woman again.

> I think this phase in your life makes you stop and think, could I have done more?

I did find that Baroness Warsi again. The fog did clear. The worst time I had it for was a period of about six weeks to two months. So I've been quite lucky that they've been short bursts – but there were two months of it at one time that I found incredibly hard to fight through and sometimes I have just had to accept "defeat" and write the day off.

For example, I have suffered from menstrual migraines all my life. And although my migraines have become less regular, when I do have them, they are more extreme. It is linked to this hormonal change. I assume there must be such a thing as menopausal migraines.

I'm not on HRT – no medication at all. I'm just trying to power through with being healthy. From the conversations I've had with doctors, and particularly my GP, I got the impression that medication wasn't going to fix it. It was just going to pause it, and at some point, I was going to have to go through this. And that if I did go on HRT there would be some level of symptoms when I came off, so I took the view, rather in my forties than my fifties or my sixties.

I think this phase in your life also makes you stop and think, could

I have done more? One of the things for me has been the Black Lives Matter movement. I grew up in a time when there was a coming of age with race relations. The Race Relations Act was passed, we thought things were getting better, the whole Cool Britannia thing as we approached the Blair era. And now I look at the Black Lives Matter movement and the rise of nationalism and nativism and – like a lot of people my age – I find myself saying, "What did we achieve?" I do think it's a symptom of this part of your life that you think: What did I actually achieve? Did it make a difference?

I had some friends over at Christmas, girlfriends from school, and we focused a lot on what we had achieved, and I remember telling them that I thought I had one big career left in me yet. One of them turned around and said, "What the hell? You've had four careers so far. Why do you feel there's another career left in you?" I think it is important to take stock.

I think this new stage has got to be: how do you become a nurturer? How do you create the space and conditions for other, younger people to fight the battles with the energy that they've got? How do you create that soft landing for people as they navigate bumpy roads? How do you do that wraparound stuff? That includes the mentoring, opening your black book, giving advice and providing opportunities for workplace experiences.

I do feel very connected with the young people involved in BLM, predominantly because my husband and I have five kids between us who are all in their twenties. They are that generation who are going to the protests, while getting their first jobs, trying to get onto the property ladder. We see the struggle they are facing. My daughter does not believe as a woman of colour that she is any less than any person who is white and she doesn't feel she is any less than any man, and why should she?

What I realise is that my daughter's expectations are higher and rightly so – they demand absolute equality for women and women of colour. And part of the responsibility we owe them is to have this conversation about the menopause, this thing that they will reach in their life, to make it less taboo so that when they hit it they're not going to have to hide it, be ashamed of what they are going through or feeling less of a woman because of it. It's about women of our age rising to their expectations and making them realise that as they hit menopause, the best years of their lives are not over, they are still ahead of them.

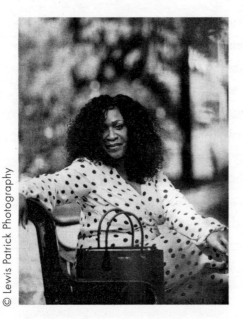

Angie Greaves

Radio host

"Menopause is as much the beginning of something as it is the end."

Angie Greaves is Smooth Radio's *Smooth Drive Home* presenter. In the late 1980s she worked at Capital Radio, where her voice was discovered, and she went on to host the Breakfast Show on Choice FM, London's first Black radio station.

~

The menopause is such a taboo subject, but I don't think we live in that much of a taboo world anymore. Age is no longer significant and at one time it was said that you should never ask a woman her age because a woman who tells you her age will tell you anything. Now, when someone asks, "How old are you?" my answer is, "Does it really matter anymore?"

And who says the menopause is for a woman in her fifties? A dear friend of mine in the States went through it at twenty-eight and now can't have children.

So, let's erase this image of the sad old woman. The default image of a woman who had gone through the menopausal process is so negative, we've been programmed to imagine a hunch-backed wrinkled female with grey hair, a bun on her head, dressed in black and lightning coming down on her. My God, no – that's not the 2020 image. Not at all.

I call the menopause Puberty Part Two. It's very, very simple: Puberty Part One, you start your periods, Puberty Part Two, you stop. I came up with that phrase because I felt that menopause sounded like something so sad, dark and final.

I remember my start of Puberty Part One, it was New Year's Day, I was eleven years of age and I went to the loo, wiped myself, saw what I saw and burst into tears. My mum said to me, "Angela, you knew this had to happen." Even though she had spoken to me about it, I still cried. Mum is quite open and simply said, "Look, we're not going to make a big thing of this. It was going to happen. It is part of becoming a woman." Then she said to me, "You've got to take your hygiene up a level," and after a really really (really) long speech she ended by saying, "And stay away from boys."

It amazes me the way that speech stays in my mind.

I hit the perimenopausal stage at about age forty-eight. The symptoms started and my eldest, who was a teenager at the time, and my youngest, who was a tweenie, found a pregnancy test in the bathroom.

"Mum's having a baby," they said.

"Erm, no," I said, "if you look closely, you'll see that the test is negative."

"So why are you taking a pregnancy test?" my eldest asked.

"Because I missed a period," was my plain and simple reply.

I didn't even think that it might be the beginning of Puberty Part Two. I had that one missed period and it wasn't until about another eight weeks that I noticed I was starting to feel really warm. I passed it off as summer warmth, as it was a really hot summer. So I bought a fan for the bedroom and it only clicked when the clocks went back and we went into autumn and winter and I was still using the fan and the penny dropped.

We really need to talk about Puberty Part Two.

Whether we're shouting about it, laughing about it or just discussing it, the topic needs to be demystified. I totally appreciate that it can be traumatic for some women who may not find the symptoms as easy to take in their stride as I did. There were a couple of occasions that I'd go out and I'd come back in and the girls would ask, "Is it raining outside, Mum?" because I would be pouring with sweat. Some mornings I would be putting my makeup on and as I applied the foundation it would be dripping off, so the fan would go on full blast. I'd just laugh, some mornings, start again and give myself extra makeup time.

What helped me big time was a six-week detox, which involved no sugar, no alcohol, no processed foods and no carbs. It was brutal at first, but that detox decreased the symptoms by about 80 per cent. I gave it another go last year, and I'm in the middle of the process now. What I do find after this detox, however, is that I can feel the effects of returning to a takeout, and especially alcohol. I'm a Prosecco fanatic, so if I do have a glass I can feel my temperature going up.

I would advise any woman to try cutting out sugar, alcohol and complex carbs – bread, potatoes, pasta, rice. Forget bread, you don't need it anyway. Basmati rice I found better than normal easy-cook rice. It was a struggle at first because on most Sundays in a Caribbean household, there'll be rice and peas, roast potatoes and macaroni cheese so I would savour Sundays for basmati rice. I personally made small changes so if I did do macaroni cheese, I went for gluten-free pasta, as brown pasta was a little heavy to digest. Potatoes were mostly replaced with chickpeas and lentils (mashed with a potato masher and a little All Purpose Seasoning. Beautiful).

Before I had these sugar-free experiences, my decision-making was affected. I did some crazy things. I couldn't find my car keys once and my girls laughed at me: "Mum, you put them in the fridge about an hour ago!" Don't ask me why. In the bathroom, I once squeezed toothpaste instead of shower gel. Now that could have been a genuine mistake, grabbing an upright toothpaste dispenser instead of the upright shower gel! But these were the things I did. The sugar alongside the raging hormones, in my opinion, causes a chemical and hormonal imbalance. Everything was an issue for me, everything was an enormous event: Shall I put my hair in a ponytail today or should I wear a wig? It would take me ages to decide. I would lay out my clothing the night before and I would get up the next day and I would change my mind.

But once I did that detox and made different choices about the foods that I digested something changed.

After research I said a flat "NO" to going on HRT. When I realised I was perimenopausal and went to the doctor, he offered me HRT, but after a bit of research I turned it down due to the cancer risk. It was a small percentage, but a risk is a risk. Also one of my friends went onto HRT and she had some severe reactions. Increased hair growth under her arms, on her arms and under her chin. She was plucking every month, not just one or two strands, and the hair seemed to appear when her period would have been due. So from HRT I steered clear.

Being of Caribbean background, my parents are very much plant-based in their medicinal approach. A story comes to mind of my first visit to Barbados. My grandad was a tall strapping man: six foot four inches and as strong as an ox. One Saturday he had flu-like symptoms, which upset me, as on the Sunday he was meant to take me to the beach. I got really upset and I said, "Grandad, if you're sick you can't take me to the beach tomorrow?" He laughed and sent me to a plant he had in his garden, which in Barbados is called the Wonder World Bush. I got him the three leaves, he squeezed the juice of the leaves, added some fresh lemon juice, a little bit of salt and a dash of Mount Gay Rum and the following day he was driving us all to the beach and swimming out to the horizon. I'm not knocking the pharmaceutical methods, but there's something to be said of natural plant-based remedies, which is why I've also become quite interested in essential oils, because the majority of them are from plants. Even my mother, who had her appendix out as a small child, was given a plant-based concoction that numbed her abdomen and dazed her.

I've now become aware of what my mum was going through when she hit Puberty Part Two. Didn't know it at the time, but boy do I see it now. Her mood swings were fierce. She'd go upstairs happy as Larry and come back down ready for action: "Who put that there?", "Who did that?", "Why are you laughing?" It was so bad I started going back to church – I thought something was wrong with me. She was probably frustrated that her Bajan herbal and plant remedies weren't available here in the UK and that probably added to the chemical imbalance. Her mood swings were awful, frightening, but still I doubt she would have taken HRT – that wouldn't have been her thing.

I've had the challenge of looking after teenagers and elderly parents. And it is a strain, big time, but it is what it is. In March 2019, because my mum is in her mid-eighties, I moved to live nearer to her; it was important and it was the right thing to do. Who saw lockdown coming exactly twelve months later? I can't imagine the stress I would have gone through had I not moved.

So I find myself with my mum being on her own at eighty-seven, my two daughters who are going on nineteen and twenty-two, and then me bang in the middle. I'm hearing from my mum, "You can't do this." And hearing from my daughters, "Oh Mum, you should do this!" So I feel caught between two generations; one saying, "Slow down a bit!" and one saying, "Let's GO!"

My mum saying, "Why do you order clothes online? Go to the shops..."

My daughters saying, "Why don't you do more online clothes shopping? It saves time, then we can go out for a drink?"

They set me clothing challenges; don't wear jeans for a week, wear more dresses, change the looks, brighten up the colours.

Then Mum would say, "Save time and money, buy one suit and loads of blouses." It's hilarious!

I love having two younger daughters who want to spend time with me, who want to do my hair, my nails, want to take charge of my wardrobe and take the edge off the fact that I'm in Puberty Part Two. My girls do keep me feeling amazing. This phase doesn't have to be a dark area that dominates your life. It can be a freeing experience.

> The phase doesn't have to be a dark area that dominates your life. It can be a freeing experience.

We had both Puberty Parts One and Two going on in the household at one time. I always know when my elder daughter's period is approaching and I duck! My younger daughter, she just takes things in her stride. She used to have very bad period pain, but that eased through essential oils. We do laugh when we do the family shop, whether in the supermarket or online: I can skip straight past the sanitary protection aisle – it's heaven.

I did have a bit of a scare a couple of years ago because I had a breakthrough bleed, so needed to be tested for cancerous cells and, with multiple fibroids shrinking, I needed a biopsy. But, thank God, all was fine.

When the phase of Puberty Part Two arrived and I knew what was happening, I thought of that conversation my mum had with me back when I was eleven... "Stop crying, you knew this had to happen." I felt the same at forty-eight and forty-nine. "Okay, you knew this had to happen..." and, oh, the freedom once I embraced that. So exhilarating.

It's about being liberated.

What a joy to have one less thing to think about! One less area of monthly stress.

What an absolute joy to go swimming, knowing you're never going to have an accident!

What an absolute joy to wear a lovely pair of white linen pants in the summer and not worry!

No cramps in the middle of the month!

I'm just loving this time. It's great.

And, since I got a hold on the sugar, which I'm convinced is a type of drug, I sleep better, my skin is clearer and there is this sense of ease.

For me, the breakdown of oestrogen can make you feel stronger. And a little increase in Vitamin D helps your bones, which do need assistance as you get older. Puberty Part Two really isn't that much of an issue today, as it was in my mother's day. There's nothing to whisper about. The forty-five to sixty demographic is rocking right now! We don't have to stop because society says that once you're of a certain age you're no longer bankable.

Menopause is as much the beginning of something as it is the end. It's like a rebirthing of the second part of your youth. It's definitely not the end.

You know, when I was young, I'd go out and see somebody my parents' age and think, *What are they doing here?* Whereas my kids come out with me. My eldest, since we're around the same size, is always asking, "Can I borrow your blouse?" or "Can I borrow that jumper?" I went out for dinner one evening with a friend and my youngest was in town and she came to the restaurant (uninvited) and helped herself to our meal. We just laughed. I would never have done that with my mother; she probably wouldn't have gone out for dinner! There are barriers that are breaking down that are bringing us closer to our kids. So why can't we bring down this barrier of Puberty Part Two?

I feel much more attractive in my fifties because I am what I am. I don't have to try. I've nothing to prove.

I took my girls to a festival a few years ago; we were in a tent with a DJ playing and I was just having a boogie with myself in the corner. My daughters were on the dance floor going for it, and one of the guys dragged me onto the dance floor – which I found quite funny. What was even funnier was that my daughters didn't cringe!

But that had to do with me feeling good in myself and not trying.

It's not just about makeup, it's not just about the hair, the ponytail or the wig, it's not just about clothing. It's about feeling good inside and that shows up on the outside.

There really is nothing to prove to anybody. Looking after yourself and putting yourself first in a healthy way is the most important thing you can do. If I don't look after myself, if I burn myself out – who is going to be there for my girls?

I so embraced menopause by calling it Puberty Part Two. I got to grips with it and got over that initial hump. I stopped stressing about it, found my coping mechanisms, and it gradually became fine. By combining positive thoughts, a healthy lifestyle and relaxation techniques, I feel like I've changed the menopause experience for myself.

I think it's about just accepting that life is what it is. It doesn't have to be the worst time EVER. Attitude makes all the difference!

I'm doing my best to be aware and present during each and every moment. Practising mindfulness prevents me from worrying about the future (which is often anxiety filled), or dwelling on the past and regret.

The Puberty Part Two time of life can be so fulfilling. We've spent many years focusing on our children, partner, or career. During menopause, we have plenty of time to think about ourselves, and rediscover who we are. Instead of viewing it as a negative time, why not try viewing it as puberty, only in reverse without the sanitary protection and cramps?

GRIEF

(noun)

Intense sorrow, especially caused by the loss
of something or someone much beloved.

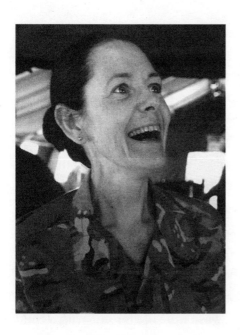

Andrea Macfarlane

RAF officer

"The threat of the menopause went to the back of my mind because I was so ill."

Squadron Leader Andrea Macfarlane, 47, is diversity and inclusion lead in the RAF. She forged a career in the army, as a rare thing in the forces then – a single mum. But in her late twenties she was diagnosed with head and neck cancer. The treatment she had for it would bring on early menopause. She has recently been part of the process of creating a menopause policy for the RAF and the Ministry of Defence.

~

I had an early menopause brought on by cancer treatment.

When I was in my late twenties I was diagnosed with stage four head and neck cancer. I'd had my daughter, Alanna, when I was in my early twenties and she was probably about seven when we found out. I remember that when I was told about the effects of chemo – I was treated between my pituitary and thyroid – there was no insight into the psychological effects of this from the all-male doctors. If I hadn't already had my daughter and it hadn't been stage four, there perhaps would have been some consideration of freezing eggs or having that option. But it was found too late and I had a three per cent chance of survival.

I had already left my job in the army because I was unwell and they thought it was stress, that it was all too much. I was in the army as a linguist at the time. I'd done a couple of detachments while my daughter was little. I'd been away a bit. It was difficult because it wasn't really the done thing to be a single mum in the army at the time. It was only just before that, in 1995, that a key naval case had gone through and a single mother had been allowed to stay in the navy – and so I was lucky I was allowed to stay.

I was counselled that perhaps it wasn't the life for me, with a child on my own. On my first detachment they took away my family allowance because they couldn't see how it worked because she was being looked after by family. Fortunately, it's much better for women in the army now.

I liked my job, but we had moved six times by the time my daughter was two. So it probably was really stressful and what I started to get was really bad headaches, which were put down to stress.

A couple of years down the line, I realised that I was properly sick. Because it said on my notes that I was stressed and it was work related, doctors didn't really take me seriously, so I ended up having to pay privately to get the diagnosis. My doctor referred me for acupuncture and the woman I was seeing for acupuncture said, "There's more to this. You need to persist with this."

When I got the diagnosis, I was really upset and I remember at the time thinking, I'm in my mid-twenties and this is it for me. I was in a relationship then and was going to get married and he just did not cope at all with not having the prospect of a family ahead. I totally get the reasons for that – and you can't hold on to somebody. If that isn't somebody's life plans, then that's it. So, unfortunately that didn't go ahead and that was a bit sad, but I had bigger fish to fry at the time.

I remember that period of being told that I was likely to go through the menopause and my relationship breakdown as a result. We just didn't have time for freezing eggs or anything. We had an operation one week, they found the cancer, and then I was in having chemo the next Tuesday. It was too quick, I get it, my life was more important. But it's really difficult to have an argument with a male doctor who can't see the emotional side of that. Probably I needed counselling, too, at the time to help me.

Important glands which regulate your whole body were radiated in the treatment. I lost so much weight because the radio and chemo together are horrific. I think the weight dropping off became the main focus because without your weight there is no sustenance there to help your body recover. And that was the biggest problem we faced in my recovery.

My thyroid went wonky as well and never recovered. So the whole thing became masked in this mess of what that treatment does to you. The threat of the menopause went to the back of my mind because I was so ill. There was nothing else other than survival and trying to eat enough to keep going. I remember lying sick, collapsed on pavements and floors. I was wearing a mask to go out before everyone was doing it for Covid-19, because I was so sick. I did two terms of home schooling with my daughter because we couldn't afford for infection to come in.

My family were fab, but I couldn't talk to them about this prospect of the menopause and how my body was changing. That was because our focus was absolutely on me being able to survive the treatment.

That loss is insignificant compared to the fact you're still here. The treatment itself is so horrific and the people around you who love you put all their energy into helping you survive and at the end of it you sort of drop off a cliff edge. Everybody is so exhausted from supporting you and I had so many difficulties maintaining friendships and family bonds at the end. Because everybody is exhausted and you've changed. It's so traumatic that your world-view is changed by the end of it and you have to reconcile what's changed for you as you go into this different life. Aspects of your fundamental being and character change as a result of going through something so different. So some friendships don't survive. Some do and in the middle of it some friends appear who weren't friends before and weren't after.

The menopause actually didn't come for me till much later. I guess I was in recovery and it wasn't until maybe five or six years later that I started to get symptoms of perimenopause and it became really evident what I was going through.

I think my periods disappeared when I went under about six stone, but as soon as my weight started creeping back on everything went back to normal. And it was the thyroid that went wonky first – because it had been radiated and it was unhappy. So all those levels started changing – and that's exhausting and knocks your energy. But there was no follow-up. I felt embarrassed about talking to anybody about it.

I would probably have been about mid-thirties and my daughter, Alanna, was about thirteen, and just nobody wanted to talk to me about it. When I brought it up it was like, "What did you expect? It was one of the things we thought might happen." I asked for my bloods and vitamins to be checked because I was exhausted. My iron count was low, but my calcium count was low as well and the doctor just put me on tablets, never thinking it could be related to the menopause.

I didn't think about the menopause because it didn't happen immediately and in the first three years I was just so excited about life, and having my mobility back – my mobility had dropped as well, as some of my nerves had been damaged. So being able to be active became a big focus. There were so many big things I was focused on that the menopause went to the bottom of the list.

Then, when it started, I was in a new relationship and I went into full panic mode. I was so embarrassed to talk about it. Nobody talked about it then. This was over ten years ago and there was very little on the internet about it either. The doctors would be like, "So what?" I wasn't offered HRT and I don't know if I would have taken it anyway.

I didn't talk about it, not to anybody, not to my partner. The problem with that was that I was in such a horrible place and the relationship broke down because I didn't cope. We'd had a fabulous relationship up until that point. It was really difficult because I hid this for years and it was so tough. There were massive blood clots that were a huge issue for me and the regulation of temperature was horrific. Also there were these pains in my bones, which were obviously to do with lack of calcium. And not being able to talk – not really knowing what were symptoms and what weren't – was a problem.

I was completely exhausted to the point that sometimes I was so tired I couldn't speak. I would get to the point where my body was just shutting down. I was in mid conversation with people in the middle of the day at work and I wouldn't be able to speak. It was like this veil that came over me and it was like the whole world greyed out. It was like that feeling when you're on a bus and you close your eyes and you're asleep. It was uncontrollable. There wasn't anything I could have done to snap out of that.

It was horrific and scary as well. Having been through cancer, when the blood clots arrived, I went into panic mode. I thought, Oh my God, what if this is something coming back?

I went to the doctor who referred me right away to have some scans and to have some bloods done to check – but who never mentioned the menopause. I said, "Could I talk about my endocrine, what my body is going through, my bloods?" And it was like, again, "Yeah, but you surely must have expected this?"

Mentally I found it really challenging because it was this whole panic about what my body was going through. The worry that the cancer had come back and that was what was causing everything. The worry that the tiredness would never go away. It did feel as though this was going to be my life from then forward.

"Why don't we support people to think about the menopause differently?

I'm currently working in diversity and inclusion, and I've just been working on the menopause policy for the RAF. One of the women from career management got in touch with me about the menopause when I first got into the post and we put stuff down and we sort of moulded it into a policy. It was going to be a leaflet, but I've just got an email back from the woman who owns the policy saying that it's going to be proper defence policy. It's not just going to be for the air force. So ours has led the way. I'm really pleased about that.

What we focused on was how we need to make adaptations based on what the individual person is experiencing – so it was more about having a person-centred approach, because everybody's different. And being able to enable the person to work in an environment that supports their needs. To be tolerant of that.

One of the things I really wanted in there was that somebody might not know what's happening to them, because it could happen at any time in somebody's life and that then gets difficult to address. How do you have that conversation? How do you as a male middle-aged manager, or even a young manager, raise something like that if you think that's what someone is experiencing? If you've got a little bit of insight into it, how do you raise it without getting your head bitten off? Especially for someone who hasn't had a family, this might be devastating for them.

Doing what I'm doing now, I do feel fortunate to have gone through the illness, because the whole process of that does bring out different sides to your character. It's really difficult at the time and it makes you into this weird, angry person for a while, but I've then been able to harness some of that and use that to help me relate to people's lived experiences. At least now I can say, "I'm able to relate to how difficult that must have been based on some of the things I've been through." Of course, it's different – the difficulties for them in their journey. It's valuable to share and that's why things like this are important.

The menopause, for me, was a whole challenge to how you see yourself and your worth as a woman. I don't think anybody talks about that properly. Our society is what it is and, of course, we challenge it, but there's something quite deep rooted, especially where I'm from. I'm from a mining community in Scotland that isn't very wealthy. It's rooted in the idea that you get married and have your children and that's it. That's the natural progression. Especially in the 1970s when I grew up. And where is it now, my identity, if this isn't who I am anymore?

Interestingly, I had another relationship a few years ago and one of the reasons it didn't progress was that he wanted children. Right at the beginning I said that isn't an option for me. It was really hurtful. I felt that relationship was taken away from me because of what I had been through, which was no fault of my own.

I was so fortunate in my friendship group at that time, because sometimes our friendships are quite transient – and the person was in our group as well. But at that moment our group was solid. I was really lucky it wasn't just my perspective that was being listened to, it was his as well. It did help me through it. That friendship group didn't just physically put their arms round me but put their arms round me metaphorically. They and my daughter, who is amazing, helped me through it. I can talk to Alanna about anything. Because she's so solid underneath.

The menopause and the end of my fertility did make me feel useless. I felt I was dumped on a scrapheap.

Why don't we support people to think about the menopause differently? Why don't we support them to manage situations like the one I was in? If I'd been better supported to manage the initial situations, when these conversations were happening right at the beginning of the relationship when the bonds were starting, I probably could have handled that a bit better – for both of us.

I'm now part of the LGBT+ community and consider myself pansexual. This wasn't something that happened overnight but was something I didn't understand until postmenopause (it was illegal to express non-heterosexuality in the military when I joined). The community has been amazingly supportive and I've found speaking to all genders about their experiences of life transition has been a powerful leveller to help me find purpose in my context.

There was no big revelation or realisation; it was a gradual understanding of who I was and how all my relationships were based on emotional connection. I had been rejecting who I was for so long, it had become a habit. But I think coming through the menopause meant that so much had changed for me and I came to see my identity as part of the bigger picture of my next chapter in life. That loss of who I thought I was, which I felt after my illness and subsequent menopause, became part of finding a way forward. It's taken over a decade for me to get through it and come to terms with how I'd like to live this next part of my life.

I think the whole journey with cancer and early menopause buried my identity further than the conformity I'd experienced growing up and in the military environment. I felt it was about survival rather than who I was.

I think now, at least, there are more resources out there. I remember desperately googling things to cope, embarrassed to be googling them, clearing my search history – now there are way more resources and openness. You're no longer, with hushed tones, saying the word "menopause". Or, "I'm going through the change." I hate that. Say what it is.

People are also talking about the more gruesome stuff that comes with it because we need to know. We need to tell people. We need to know that actually you do get a version of baby brain because hormones affect your ability to retain information, to regulate your time. I went through a period of not being able to get to meetings at the right point or right time. It affects your whole being – and being able to talk about that is so helpful.

When I went through the cancer treatment people didn't say the word "cancer" either. It was seen as a death sentence. It was right at the beginning of bringing awareness to it – the Race For Life had just started at that point. Having been through that journey, perhaps it better prepared me for this. Because that was something hidden and then people started talking about it, and the whole social inclusion campaign around that probably gave me some insight into the things that need to be done to move forward on this – and I don't think we're anywhere near it.

When you go through the menopause early you do feel really lonely because you see it as an old person's thing. And it's been really important to me to be able to write a policy that's inclusive of age – to include the fact that somebody young might be going through this and not be able to approach what that means for them.

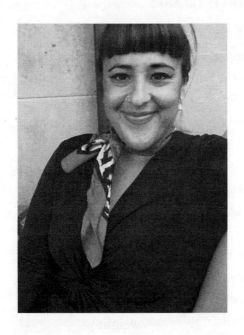

Sahira Ahmad Belcher

Fire service official

"My periods stopping made me feel old — like I was not quite part of the group anymore."

Sahira Ahmad Belcher, 45, is an official for the Oxfordshire fire service. She began her perimenopausal symptoms not long after the birth of her daughter, Indy. She was just thirty-five and it took a four-year battle for her to get a diagnosis. She suffered depression and still now, on HRT, she struggles with anxiety.

~

I had an early menopause. I'm forty-five now and it's been going on for ten years and still hasn't finished yet. Sometimes I think, Please just go. I don't want to wait anymore.

The symptoms started the year I had Indy, my daughter. My periods became irregular and some months I wouldn't have a period at all. I'd also have the hot flushes and just be really anxious and sad all the time, really down.

I went to the doctor who said, "Oh, it's your hormones because you've just had a child. It will calm down." But it continued and I kept going back and forth.

It was hard after my daughter was born. The birth had been really traumatic and I had a panic attack on the table. I felt paralysed, I couldn't move and Indy was just placed there and all I was thinking was, Can someone help me?

After that I struggled to breastfeed. My milk never came in. Even at that point it felt like my hormones didn't work for me and from then on it didn't stop. I think I had a bit of postnatal depression. I knew there was something going on and that was what prompted me to do some research and find out what it was.

I was feeling totally exhausted. I had aches and pains. My sex drive was, and still is, non-existent. There was weight gain for no reason. It seemed like I had every symptom under the sun. I wasn't able to sleep and that sleep deprivation just kills you. I started to track my cycle when I had one, and I noticed that for three weeks out of a month my PMT was severe. I lacked patience. I was really irritable. My skin got really spotty. It was like I was going through puberty again. I thought, Why am I getting zits? I'm thirty-five. It's ridiculous.

With the hot flushes I wasn't sure what they were at first. I remember getting hot and thinking it was really weird because I always used to be cold all the time. I normally would have palpitations before they would come and I would think I was having some sort of heart attack. I would get really anxious. I've since been to see a consultant about getting my heart rate checked and a heart monitor, and they said, "It's just to do with your hormones."

After I'd done my own research, I knew that normally before a hot flush you can get palpitations. So I said to the doctor, "I think it's probably either perimenopause or menopause . . ."

The doctor said, "Don't be daft. It can't be that. You're far too young."

I wasn't taken seriously. I went home again. It was going round and round in my head. I was thinking, There's something wrong with me and I need someone to validate it.

It took a few years of going back and forth to get a diagnosis. I saw this one GP, an old lady, who basically said, "What are you complaining about? Pull yourself together. You should be glad you haven't got periods anymore."

At some point I saw this really good locum doctor who listened to me and said, "Look, I'm going to do a load of blood tests because it doesn't always show in your blood tests either. I'll give it a month and do another lot." The tests showed him that I was really low on everything. I was anaemic as well.

I was probably about forty when I got the proper diagnosis. It was a relief to get it. When you have all these symptoms, you start to think there are all sorts of things wrong with you. You think of all these different illnesses. I thought I might have dementia because of the brain fog – I would, and still do, forget the most basic things, forget people's names. I thought I had ME [myalgic encephalomyelitis] at one point because I was so exhausted. You work yourself up so much because you're so anxious and then finally you get the diagnosis – and that's good in some ways because it feels like it's not in your head and someone is actually taking you seriously.

It was really hard to talk about the fact I was perimenopausal. I was thirty-five. That's quite young. In my group of friends there was no one else going through it, so I felt like I couldn't really make people understand what it was like for me. And my periods stopping made me feel old – like I was not quite part of the group anymore. When you hear your friends saying they've got their period, in a weird way, you miss it. I felt a bit cheated – I'd just had my daughter and I wanted to enjoy that time more, but I was having all these symptoms. I felt it wasn't fair – why did it have to happen? I knew it would eventually, but it just happened too soon.

There was a point when I hit rock bottom. I remember my husband taking me to the doctor and the doctor saying, "Yeah, it looks like you're menopausal and you've got anxiety and depression."

I was put on antidepressants and the doctor signed me off work. I used to be really against going on any medication, but I needed them. I was off work for about six months because I just couldn't function. I was so exhausted. I didn't go back to the job I'd been in, working for a charity – there hadn't been much support there. Instead I went to work in the fire service and that's where I'm working now. Subsequently the fire service has set up a support group, but there are still no policies in place – and that's what I would really like to see. I'd like to see policies in all workplaces.

The symptoms aren't so bad now because I'm on HRT – and testosterone gel as well. It's helping, but I feel like I need more adjustments; it's not a one-size-fits-all either. I've been on and off and on and off the antidepressants. When Covid-19 first hit, my anxiety was through the roof. I managed to speak to the GP and she prescribed the antidepressants again. I've been all right since then, but it's very up and down. It's just an absolute nightmare really.

I eventually want to come off the antidepressants because I don't know what's working and what isn't at the moment. People say if you're on the right HRT you won't need the antidepressants.

I don't know why I had the menopause that early. My mum didn't have hers until she was fifty. I've got two sisters and my sister who is going to be fifty next year is only starting to get peri now. The other one is going to be forty and she's not had any symptoms either. I've wondered if there might be a link with the fact that I did have quite a traumatic birth and a caesarean. There is also supposed to be a link between low birth weight and early menopause. That theory's interesting to me because I was a twin.

Even now people assume I'm not at the menopause, because they associate it with someone a lot older. I think people need to realise that it does affect younger women. You hear of teenage girls going through it, and women who have had cancer treatment. The lack of support out there is just abysmal.

> I often feel really sad for my daughter because I feel like she's missed out on the cheerful happy me I used to be.

But no one should suffer in silence. What we need is more education of GPs, proper teaching in mainstream schools, policies in the workplace. Because doctors often don't take you seriously, you need to keep pushing to be taken seriously. It took five years for me to get diagnosed. You shouldn't have to fight for it. They should listen to you and do the tests.

It's got to be taught at school because every woman is going to go through this and everyone needs to have some idea of what it's like. Things have got to change. I can see on the online support groups that there are a lot of women suffering. They feel like they're not being taken seriously or they're being fobbed off. It really shouldn't happen.

It's so important that workplaces have policies in place. You don't want to be penalised if you're feeling really fatigued. You don't want to be penalised if you wake up and realise, Oh my God, I literally cannot function and need to take a day off.

I joined a lot of support groups for the menopause. When I first joined some at thirty-five, it was mainly women in their fifties going through it. And it was a bit weird for me because there was no one my age raising a little baby at the same time and struggling. It was really hard to identify with anyone.

I had wanted to have other children, but obviously the menopause put a spanner in the works. Recently I found myself getting really clucky – so we got a puppy. I'm mothering a puppy now, so that feels good!

Sometimes you feel guilty because you feel you've changed as a person as well. I often feel really sad for my daughter because I feel like she's missed out on the cheerful happy me I used to be. I was always so happy-go-lucky, and now I get grouchy and tired and my patience is really low. She never got to meet the person who I used to be – and you grieve for that as well.

I felt a whole loss of identity. I have definitely changed as a person. I did see a counsellor who said I shouldn't beat myself up about it because my daughter didn't know what I was like anyway. But you do grieve for your old self.

I was making two transitions at once – firstly to being a mother, but also to being a menopausal woman. It's quite traumatic, isn't it? You get a bit angry and a bit bitter. You go through all these emotions, but obviously you have to accept it, you've got no choice. But you still feel bitter about it. Really there is no rhyme or reason for it. Why did it happen so soon?

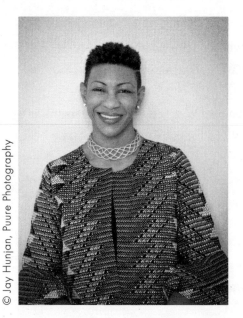

Yvonne John

Service manager,
photographer and
childlessness campaigner

*"How I interact, how I see
myself, how I allow myself to
be seen is very different from
how I was ten years ago and
I'm very excited."*

Yvonne John, 49, is a haematology service manager. After she married, aged thirty-nine, she and her husband tried for three years to have a baby. The grief and self-blame when that didn't happen were feelings she would later process when she joined Gateway Women. She went on to write a book, *Dreaming of a Life Unlived: Intimate stories and portraits of women without children*, and become a campaigning voice and activist for childless women of colour.

~

I only realised recently that I must be perimenopausal when I took a look at the list of symptoms and saw I had quite a few of them. Also I talked to a friend, who is also forty-nine. We're the same age, and she said, "We must be in the perimenopause, just because of our age."

I'm childless not by choice (CNBC). I tried to conceive naturally for three years, with my husband, during my early forties. My relationship with my periods changed during that time because not only were they painful and heavy, as they had always been, but I had grown to really hate them in a different way. Every month they were a reminder that trying to conceive didn't work. It was a reminder of what my body wasn't doing – of not having that dream you were dreaming of, your hopes being dashed. I think it made the whole experience of having a period a lot worse; it was telling me month after month that there was no baby.

It brought a little grief during each cycle, a layer of sadness. Previously, because my periods were bad, I had the experience of thinking, "Crap, I'm on my period," but I would kind of get on with it. Over the years, you learn to manage it as best you can. But when it came to trying to conceive, every month you are hoping it worked, you are hoping you're pregnant and then your body tells you, "No, not this time." My period's arrival would be about absorbing the fact that it didn't happen this time.

It was often really difficult to sit with my husband, the person who I loved and wanted a family with, and not be able to see that desire be fulfilled. As the years went on, it got harder and harder and I got angrier and angrier. There was more arguing around it because you just have this urgency and this desperation. It's got to be this time. It's got to work. We've got to try harder. Forget kissing, forget foreplay, let's just get on with it.

It became the most robotic experience – horrible. And you feel, in a way, you are dragging someone else through it because no one chooses to go through that. The anger, the emotions that get involved! No one signs up for that. And even if you think it might be hard you're not prepared for how hard it actually is.

I didn't know that what I was feeling was grief until an older (CNBC) friend told me that I was grieving and introduced me to

Jody Day from Gateway Women. At first I felt I didn't deserve to grieve, because there was a lot of self-blame and shame for me. I did Gateway Women's year-long Plan B mentorship programme, which saved my sanity and helped me to reconcile my feelings. I felt like not being able to conceive had to be my fault because in my twenties I had two terminations. I felt that people would judge me and would say that I didn't deserve to be here if they knew about my past.

I decided to write a book about childlessness. At first I thought I shouldn't include the story of my terminations in it. I remember being invited to speak at my first event and saying to the woman who organised it, "If you knew my whole story you wouldn't ask me to speak." I told her about the terminations and she said, "So what?"

I recently had a hysterectomy. I had very painful heavy periods in my thirties and I found that in my forties it got a lot worse. I've been wondering if that might have been because of the perimenopause, but no one properly talked to me about that. I read some blurb around irregular periods and thought, *I wonder*. I remember years ago, in my thirties, a GP said, "Maybe it's your age." I really wanted to slap him after hearing that.

I got to the place where I couldn't function without painkillers. It was so bad I'd feel I would have to overdose on painkillers just to have some normality in terms of not feeling the pain. Also the heavy bleeding and my anxieties around that was crazy. I'd be in meetings thinking about it, wondering if I had leaked, worrying about the blue chair I was sitting on. I noticed, in the last year or two, it started to get more erratic, and would sometimes come a week earlier, or it would die down and I would think I'm on a light day, and then it would just flood. There were even times where I'd have to clean the chair in a restaurant.

I've had fibroids as well and I did end up in front of different

consultants telling me, "Your only option is to have a hysterectomy."
I was in floods of tears and my only thoughts were, Hell no. I'm not
doing that. I couldn't reconcile losing my womb at that point.

That was the beginning of this three-year journey of being
around consultants. A different consultant decided to arrange an
MRI, because she said that sometimes people are misdiagnosed with
fibroids, and she wanted to check. She then found out I did have
fibroids, but also adenomyosis, which is similar to endometriosis.
They call it the evil twin to endometriosis. It was the cause of the
pain and heavy bleeding. I found out then that could have contributed to me not being able to conceive a child as well.

They said the only cure for me was a hysterectomy. I remember a
friend telling me, "Think of it as losing the pain, not as losing your
womb, and as getting your life back."

What I kept thinking was that I hated my womb because it didn't
do what I wanted it to do and allow me to conceive.

I had this whole journey of trying to reconcile my grief around
childlessness, my anger towards my womb and the need to have a
better quality of life. Therapy really helped me to have that space
to talk and work through all my feelings, including writing a letter
to say goodbye to my womb. In that letter I expressed all the anger
and the hurt I had around it. That really helped to verbalise it all and
kind of put it in a place where I wasn't so hurt by it. I was then able
to be in a place where I was like, "Okay, I can do this now."

I did expect to feel really crap after the hysterectomy. I expected
to be in floods of tears and grieving about it, but I think because
I had done all my grieving before I had the surgery, and had said
goodbye to my womb, as it was such a conscious decision to do it,
I just felt relief. I just felt at peace with it because I was able to say
goodbye; I had already done my crying. And I was then in a place
of recovery and I could go away and have the space to just recover.

In terms of perimenopausal symptoms I have short-term memory loss, for sure. I can forget things within seconds of being told. I'll be having conversations and I'll be like, what's the word for something? I just cannot remember it. I have breast tenderness. I have urinary urgency and I've started to have night sweats as well. But that's very recent.

I didn't recognise these as perimenopausal symptoms until I looked them up; it really shows how little this is talked about.

> Talking to other people about all I've been through has made me realise that all this shit is normal.

Most of these symptoms I had I thought were just because of my age, especially regarding the memory loss. Even weight gain; again, I remember people were always saying that in your forties you will find it harder to lose weight. Finding out that I am perimenopausal just made me realise what my body's telling me, which I did actually know before but I can still quite easily forget, that I am this age. This is my body telling me, "No, you really are forty-nine."

In my Caribbean culture, I find — and I'm sure African cultures are quite similar — that there isn't much conversation around periods and the menopause. You seem to have to find out about these things on your own or from your friends. I remember the mention of Aunt Flo visiting, when referring to your period, or the fact that someone is "going through the change" when referring to the menopause. It's almost like the words *period* and *menopause* are too shameful to mention let alone talk about.

I think all that I've been through has made me realise how little people talk about things and how little an understanding we have of what our bodies are actually going through. You can go to the GP or have a symptom of something and it seems to be treated in isolation.

No one is looking at the whole picture. No one's connecting what's happening throughout your whole body.

I feel I can talk about almost anything now. Talking to other people about all I've been through has made me realise that all this shit is normal. There's such a taboo around absolutely anything and everything about women's bodies that you just don't realise that, actually, this is life. This is normal. Everyone's going through something and there's no release or healing around it until you do.

One of the things I remember thinking when I was trying to have children was I didn't want to hit the menopause and not have tried. I remember thinking, I've got to try because if I hit my menopause and I hadn't tried, I would have seriously regretted it. I've since given a lot of talks because of my involvement with Gateway Women and am very aware that with all the stories around women's fertility journeys, people only want to hear the ones that end in a miracle baby.

When you are struggling to have a child, people always want to keep you in this state of hope and denial and "let's try and fix it for you". I think this is one of the difficulties for childless women going through the menopause.

I co-facilitate the Gateway Women Reignite Weekend workshops where I've heard stories around women regarding the menopause or being perimenopausal. For many women who have been on the childless journey for a number of years, I think the menopause brings up a different layer of grief around childlessness because now they are truly at the end of their fertility journey.

But my journey isn't like that. I dealt with the grief of childlessness before I got to the stage of menopause. My trigger wasn't the menopause or being perimenopausal, but I'm aware I don't know how I will feel when I hit the menopause itself. However, my finality of not having children has already hit me. I don't have a womb anymore, so in a sense I have already recognised that as the end of my journey to conceiving my own child. I couldn't have done it without the support of my Gateway sisters or my therapist, along with writing the letter to say goodbye to my womb. I had the space to grieve with someone holding my hand through it. So I feel fortunate in that sense.

I'm actually really excited about becoming fifty because, for me, my forties represented my fertility journey and the grief and sadness around it. That's over now in terms of no longer sitting in hope anymore. I'm no longer actively trying to have a baby. It's not going to happen. So, this is the new phase of my life. I feel like forty-nine is reinventing myself and at fifty I'm going to come out of the cocoon; I'm a butterfly.

I see my fifties being about rediscovering me and looking forward to living up to my full potential. It's no longer being afraid. It's being free. It's experiencing anything and everything about me. It is being fearless.

I'm separated and divorcing, and I am excited about dating. For me, the mindset of dating is so different now, going into my fifties, because it's not about getting married and having kids. It's so different how I interact with men now. I feel freer. I think I'm going to grow old disgracefully. Dating doesn't matter in the way that it did when I wanted to be married, when I was looking for my life partner and the man I'm going to have kids with, there was all that pressure around finding the right one. There is now a freeness around it because I'm not looking for a husband and not going to have children. How I interact, how I see myself, how I allow myself to be seen is very different from how I was ten years ago and I'm very excited.

I've accepted myself now. I'm like if you want to be around me, be here, if you don't, don't. I never really felt like that before. My whole definition of relationships has changed. I do not really believe in the happy-ever-after like I did in the past.

In dealing with the grief I felt I had to really redefine a lot of things that I believed in – religion, marriage, that "happy-ever-after" story. I had to understand why I was led to believe that I was going to be and should be a mum because it hurt so much when I didn't get the fairy-tale ending. The same when my marriage broke up, I had to understand what all that meant to me and what it would mean for me in the future. I had to redefine what it all meant because if I didn't do that, I wouldn't have survived.

I don't ever remember anyone telling me there was an option not to have kids or that it may not happen. With the family members who don't have kids – and there are some – there was no recollection of hearing about their lives. I only remember hearing about those key milestones; yes, you heard that someone was getting married but the excitement was always about someone being pregnant, the birth of a child (because the family was growing), or someone becoming a grandparent.

One of the things I've realised is that I've had to create my own milestones. If I'd had children the next stage would have been grandchildren, but I'm on my own. So I have to come up with my own milestones, like turning fifty and becoming this badass woman. I'm on version 2.0 now, so what's the next version of me going to look like? What's the postmenopause me going to look like?

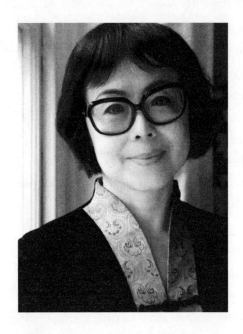

Xinran Xue

Author

"We are all part of it. In family life, everybody is part of it. In the whole society, everyone is part of it. You can't chop off the hands and say the hands need to be improved."

Xinran Xue, 62, grew up in China and moved to London in 1997. When she was growing up, her parents were imprisoned during China's cultural revolution. As an adult, living in China, she presented a radio show called *Words on the Night Breeze*, which focused on women's life stories. She later moved to the UK and began menopausal symptoms during a period in which her husband was diagnosed with cancer. Her books include *The Good Women of China*, *Messages from an Unknown Chinese Mother* and *The Promise: Love and Loss in Modern China*.

~

I gave birth to my son quite late compared to most Chinese, at thirty years old. So when I started the menopause my son was a teenager, in puberty. And in China we say the most difficult, hard time is when the mother has the menopause and the children are teenagers. That's exactly what happened to me. Also, around then, my husband discovered he had cancer – and he would later die from cancer in 2017.

In fact, I didn't have time to think much about my feelings. I couldn't allow myself to be moody. I had hot flushes, and I noticed something wrong with my period but I had no time for it, because of my family's needs and my worldwide book tours, but most especially my son, who started talking in a very sharp language – spicy and chilli in black and white! – including lots of chat about girlfriends and he even asked me the very big question, "What is a woman?"

My son sometimes said, "You're very, very Chinese." But for me I always thought, No, I'm very different from most Chinese women. But when the menopause happened, I found I came back to being more Chinese – because in Chinese culture we never talk about physical problems and also we never talk about family – particularly for women. So in China, we would never say, "It's your first husband or second husband?" We would never say, "Is it your own child, or step-child or adopted?" We would never ever talk about this.

We would always avoid the subject. We would never talk about this kind of problem before I left China in 1997. Chinese women started talking about it from ten or less years ago. For me, I didn't even think to tell my son that I had started this kind of change or physical problem. My husband – the literary agent Toby Eady – realised I had, and he was a very kind person, he loved me, unconditionally, and he realised there was something in my books that was different. Normally my writing is very focused to the interviewee, my object, and the people in my book. In that time I think I started to put myself in more than before. I think that was very much linked to the menopause.

When I lived in China, I had a nine-year radio show, called *Words on the Night Breeze*, a bit like *Woman's Hour*. I heard about the menopause during that time, but I'd never really thought about how the women felt. I always heard it as men, or children, or parents talking about someone who had changed. I never really thought about this as a person like myself. And that time in China was very bad for any girls who thought about sex, or women who even wanted to have another look at a strange man in the street; they could be called a sexual hooligan, or even arrested for that.

In China we didn't have public sexual education or psychology education until 2003. The whole of China's 5,000-year history, we never had that. But we had a very traditional way to pass this kind of knowledge down. When you were married or engaged, you were given a box by your mother – and inside were lots of pictures and reports of this kind of knowledge of men, of sex, of babies and pregnancy. Also for the wealthy families, like my mum's, there was this special bed. And in this bed all around the top, the wooden part, a frieze ran round and you couldn't see the pictures on it from the outside, but when you lie down you can see all the pictures about how to make love. When you lay down and put the curtain down, then you would see all the pictures there.

So, in families, we had these traditions. But during the Cultural Revolution from 1966 we stopped them. We treated these things like dirty or criminal things. So, in my generation, we never had this knowledge. When I had my first period, when it started, I didn't know what it was. I was so scared. I thought my body was injured. I was in the political children's prison, and an elder girl who was like an older sister to me, told me what it was. I was so scared, before she told me, I used a plaster to stop the blood. This is why in my marriage to my English husband he was so surprised – many times, he said, "Xinran, you've had a child already, but you look like you've never been married before."

The menopause brought back memories and emotions from

childhood. I started to think more about my teenage years and my first lover and how I was when I started to think about men. I thought about the first time I physically felt loss of control. I'd never thought about this.

I also remembered how, during my radio show, when women wrote letters to me more than 90 per cent of them said they felt guilty – they talked about how bad they are, how they are bad women because they think about men and think about physical needs and want to make love. I was really shocked. All of China full of these bad women? And I realised that I'm part of that, so I started learning and studying. But in China at that time, the 1980s, it was hard to get any books. Finally I got some books from Hong Kong and Singapore about women's psychology, and I got a full course of that, and then I interviewed a psychologist.

I went back to China at the end of 2019 until February this year [2020] to do research on suicide amongst elder women in China. It's a very sad story. There was a UN report that had found that Asian women committed suicide; there had been a 500 per cent rise in the past few years. I travelled to about six different places and I could see why many widows, who outlive their husbands, were committing suicide. And now, thinking about the menopause, this made me realise why they thought of their bodies as evil – because they felt they became crazy.

In the rural countryside when a woman started experiencing the menopause changes in her fifties, the first thing they thought, many of them told me, was that their bodies were being controlled by a ghost, a spirit, and they had become evil – because they became moody and crazy and had this very strange heat.

Many of them would carry a kind of poison bottle that they had prepared. They gave me reasons, saying that they didn't have anyone to help them, and didn't want to cost their children's future

– for money or time – and they didn't have neighbours or society to help them because their villages are disappearing, swallowed up by China's rapid urbanisation. So some widows carry this bottle of poison to the mountains, and do it there, so the mountain fire-wardens would find them and bury them.

When I interviewed women in the poor countryside, some would say, "I've been consumed by evils, my body has become very strange, I'm crazy. I don't want to hurt anyone or harm anyone." Some of them cut themselves because they didn't know their body, or how to deal with it; they had never been educated.

Also, many lonely peasant women are talking to animals, they need to talk, and when they don't have a society in which to talk, when they have not been educated in knowledge about the body, when they don't have support from NGOs and an open society, they are just living in a box, lonely. So finally they would kill themselves.

My mother was like a bronze statue in my life. I only knew this very calm face, not a lot of language, and even when she talked to us it was with the use of very short sentences – hardly any adjectives or adverbs. You would just get orders from her. She always had a very bad temper and a cold voice, so my brother and I were always scared to talk to her before she was sixty-plus years old.

I never even thought I could have talked about the menopause with my mother, but we did start this conversation since my father passed away, almost the same year as my husband. We had both lost husbands. We both are living in memory of the men in my life. I think my mother started talking about the body changes. My mother had never really talked to me before and never really had a chance to be the mother in my life.

This was because like many young couples in 1950s China, my parents had to devote their time and energy to the political party and country, and would have been judged bad or selfish if they spent time with their own children. I was sent away when I was thirty days old and sent back for education when I was seven and a half, weeks before the Cultural Revolution took place. They were later arrested and jailed. Many years later when I saw them again, I was in university; we were in different cities.

Since her husband and my husband passed away, my mum has been coping. I just noticed that after sixty-five, her moods calmed down. She told me that she felt physically calmer. Lots of anger disappeared. She started thinking about motherhood, what that meant to her, and her love for us, her own children. I now talk to her every Saturday and she started expressing some sort of regrets. This menopause has maybe been a good thing to get her back to being a woman. I never felt my mother had that. Sometimes I felt maybe I was adopted because I felt my mother never had warmth, or motherhood or womanhood. But after that I think she changed.

I've also been looking after some widows in my area in London as well. Many of them are in their eighties and I've been looking after them on like a weekly, monthly thing. We have a drink, a talk, a telephone call. I discovered that 80 per cent of them still carry on their menopause symptoms. They're in their eighties. One of the ladies, Ms F, is eighty-four now and when we are very cold in autumn or spring, she's still getting hot flushes. I say, "My lady, are you okay?" She says, "Oh, I just can't get rid of these hot flushes."

I think I was about fifty-five when I had the menopause. But I really don't know because at that time my book was published and I was a butterfly going on this publicity tour round many countries; some books more than forty languages, some books more than twenty languages. So I was very busy. But these hot flushes really became quite clear around fifty-four and fifty-five.

I think it's very important that women don't feel the menopause is their individual problem, that we don't feel it's our personal fault which comes from something we did in our past. Also that we feel it is shared with other people. I can feel the safety of the system here – medical support, psychological support, and the fact that at least you can talk about it.

> I do feel freedom. I can see it in my mother as well.

Talking is important. I'm involved in this movement of talking and educating about periods, because if you don't talk about it, if you hide it, it can cause so many problems. In the past, China never had women's equal rights, because people were never educated in this way. But in China, in many cities now – in over 665 cities – the big cities, women have much more opportunities and are more educated, more open. These last few years many girls in China have held up signs in the centre of the city saying, "Let's talk about periods." I just actually had a letter from my student. She's a professor now and she said, "Do you believe that this feminist movement started from your programme? Now I realise why so many men hated you in the 1980s and 1990s."

In China at the moment the divorce situation has become very serious. If you analyse the number of divorces, there are two very big points: one is after the young couple have had a child, and the second is when the children are at university and their family duties are finished and they want time for themselves. This is their excuse. If you look at the ages, most of them are in two groups. One is between their late twenties and early thirties; another one is between forty-eight and fifty-six. So you ask them, "Why did you do it?" They say they feel for the parents, for the family, but in fact if you ask more questions about the details of daily life and about how their struggles are, you see they sleep less, sometimes they have family problems, but actually it's based on the woman changing. She feels that nobody understands her and everyone is selfish within the family. Actually it is just her body has changed.

You have devoted your life to your parents and your children. You didn't have time for yourself – and now you want some. But to be honest we start this struggle from the first period. I think women start suffering this from our periods because every month we have moods no one could understand. You're a woman, we realise, and we suffer pain, and we suffer loneliness because we can't talk about these things, because no one cares. Even your own mother doesn't care. She just gives you a hug and says, "Oh, poor thing."

One of the things I have said is that if we want an equal society between men and women, we have to talk about what happens from the first period. Then we also have to think about the menopause. Because finally we are free from this type of physical cycle and pain and family duty. Many of us want time for ourselves. In many cultures, freedom of women starts after this menopause.

I do feel freedom. I can see it in my mother as well.

I also feel I've gained freedom during the 2020 quarantine, because I don't feel a duty for anyone. I can treat myself, whatever my body wants. Before in publicity, or business, or society, you have to behave yourself for others. But sometimes when the menopause starts you can't say to people, "Sorry, I'm in this wave." Ms F, one of my widows, always does. She still says "Sorry, I can't help now" – and fans herself.

I always think the most important thing is that we educate our men. We need to educate the children how to understand and tolerate the mother, how to give a woman space to be crazy. That's very much men that need to do that, not women.

If you have a father, you learn from your father, how he treats the mother, as a family. These changes we go through in, for instance, menopause or puberty, are happening to everybody – to the boys, to the girls, to the mother, to the whole family. But we don't talk in that way. We say that it's a woman's problem, it's a boy's problem, it's a teenager's problem. No, we are all part of it. In family life, everybody is part of it. In the whole society, everyone is part of it. You can't chop off the hands and say the hands need to be improved. But our society is like this. This is why our family problems grow.

Men and boys need to be educated about women's periods, their physical changes, and then they start this kind of caring about women. They see that women, even if they are very strong, even if they are a wolf, even if they work, even if they hold the sky, they are still women.

I never cried in China, but my husband said to me, "You can cry in front of me, it's not weakness." He said, "I can cook." All these years of fighting for women's rights, we never realised these were men's problems not women's problems. Education missed, men's problems.

My doctor thought I had depression, caused by the loss. I don't feel this kind of depression now. But I feel I'm ready to join my husband – something like that. Every night I go to bed I tidy my flat, talk to nobody and just talk to my soul and say I'm ready and I want to leave a clean, nice house.

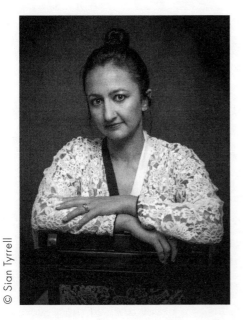

© Sian Tyrrell

Shalini Bhalla-Lucas

Author and entrepreneur

"Right now if we say we're not going to have kids, this could be it for us. I think that realisation, for me, is partly liberating. But also it's another bereavement for me."

Shalini Bhalla-Lucas, 45, is an author, entrepreneur, TV and radio presenter and the founder of Just Jhoom! – a Bollywood-inspired dance-fitness company. She is also an international mindfulness and meditation teacher. When she was forty, her husband, Jeremy, died of renal cancer and she went through a period of depression and alcohol abuse, before setting off on a series of adventures. In 2019 these took her to Kenya, where she felt the onslaught of new symptoms – hot flushes, insomnia, weight gain and mood swings.

~

When perimenopause came to me first, I experienced it as a form of grief, because I could relate it to the original grief I felt when I lost my husband, Jeremy, to renal cancer.

I'm forty-five, but I've never actually felt my age. I lived for so long with Jeremy, who was older than me, that I always felt even younger.

I started to become aware of perimenopausal symptoms recently. I was visiting a friend's house and I said, "I have to sit down. I'm feeling really hot." It wasn't a particularly hot day and I hadn't done anything strenuous – but a feeling crept up over my face. It was really weird and I went hot and cold and I thought maybe I'd eaten something bad. But it went away pretty quickly.

I realised I wasn't sleeping well, suffering from insomnia, which I have done before, because I've been through bereavement and depression, but there was no reason I should be feeling that way now. I was actually the happiest I'd been since Jeremy's death. I was also having hot flushes, and bleeding like crazy, really heavy and very painful.

I started putting all these things together. I began to have mood swings and I'm not a moody person. I'm a happy person. I practise mindfulness. I teach dance. But things were beginning to irritate me.

> It was such a shock for me because you don't think about menopause till it happens to your friends or family.

And so I called my friend Cheeku and said, "I've got all these symptoms."

She said, "Shal, do you remember when I went through perimenopause, I went through all these different symptoms? I couldn't sleep at night, hot flushes, waking up in a sweat, so similar. Shal, I think you're going through the menopause."

I said, "No, no, no, I'm forty-five. It's too early for me to be going through menopause."

I remember how when Cheeku told me she was going through menopause, it was not long since I had been bereaved from Jeremy. I just cried when she called me. She had always wanted to be a mum but never got the opportunity, and now her body was telling her she would never have children. So I felt a bereavement for her. It was such a shock for me because you don't think about it till it happens to your friends or family.

I've never wanted children. When I was sixteen, I decided I wasn't going to have kids, and when I met Jeremy at twenty-one, I didn't want kids and he already had three kids from his first marriage. That was one of the things that attracted us to each other: that I didn't have to have his kids, he didn't want to give me kids – it was perfect. But when he died, for one week I kept thinking I should have had his child, because at least I would have something of his.

That was the first time I realised that actually, I wasn't in control of having his child – when he was no longer there. Six months after he died, I set up an education fund in his name in Kenya, and now we support sixteen children through the Jeremy Lucas Education Fund. And so, for me, I now feel I have those sixteen children. I haven't had to give birth to them, but they are part of my – part of our – legacy.

But then, this started happening,

Recently I started seeing someone new, and I had this conversation with him about how he doesn't want children, and I know I don't want children. But I said to him, "You realise you could be a hundred years old and still have kids. That's not the case for me and right now if we say we're not going to have kids, this could be it for us." I think that realisation, for me, is partly liberating. But also it's another bereavement for me.

There's a contrariness to it. On the one hand, I'm like, "It's great I don't have to worry about ever having children I've never wanted." But on the other hand I'm seeing my body's actually not in my control.

So much of my life had been in what I perceived to be in my

control, then one day, Jeremy died, and I realised I had no control of anything really. And for me, going through this time of my life with perimenopause has been showing me something. Having lost my husband, having had to change my life, I'm now realising how little control I actually have. I have control of my thoughts. I have control of my reactions to certain curveballs and challenges thrown my way. But other than that I don't have any control. Part of it is liberating. Part of it is grief – and I'm in that place right now.

After Jeremy died, the first year of grief was awful. I was a recluse. There was a lot of drink and substance abuse. I abused painkillers and alcohol and food and my body. I tried to kill myself, because I didn't want to go through the bereavement. And then I started writing my book and I came out of that. That was a very cathartic process.

Then my father died eighteen months after Jeremy and I stood at his funeral, and I spoke, and I remember thinking, *I want to live again*, because both my father and Jeremy had wanted to live. They were both youngish men – Jeremy was fifty-nine, my dad was sixty-nine – and cancer had got both of them. And here I had health. I had youth. I was only forty and that's still young in today's age. I was throwing it away.

After that I decided I was going to live again. I lost weight, I got a new wardrobe, I got a personal trainer, I changed my diet, I subscribed to six dating sites in England. In seven months I spoke to fifty guys. I dated about twenty-one of them. One week I had five dates. I was out there. And then a guy hurt me and I came out of that a little bit bruised.

I realised that I had to find happiness within me, not in another man. Living in England was not serving me well. I needed to make some changes – and I had to be fearless in my decisions.

I thought, Why not just throw caution to the wind and get out there. So I learned to ride a motorbike and I bought one. I gave away three-quarters of my stuff. I rented my house out. I went to live in

London for three months so that I could spend time in a city. I went to Sri Lanka I drove a tuk-tuk around the island for two weeks. And then I came to Kenya in December 2019.

A few months later the pandemic hit. The good thing is that I met a guy here and we started going out and it was great. That's when I began to realise my body was changing. I was becoming more sexually active, and it was almost as if the next stage of my life started and I was seeing this guy, now my body was changing. The other thing that's really affecting me is I'm putting on a lot of weight. I know that's not just a lockdown thing, because I'm exercising and eating healthily. I'm very aware of my body changing, and I don't particularly like it because it's out of my control.

I'm wondering if this sex drive I've got is part of the perimenopause too. I can't get enough of it. I can't stop thinking about it.

One of the things about being an Indian woman is you are expected to have children and there are all these questions. "Why don't you have children?" and "What's wrong with you?"

Now that suddenly it feels like that choice may be being taken from me, I'm thinking, What is wrong with me? I've always thought it's my body and my life. It's my choice. Now the difference is actually it's not my choice. It's still my body, still my life, but now it's not my choice.

My story is based around dance, mental health and bereavement – and I believe that has shaped who I am and shaped and defined my body. The menopause has become part of that story. It's really interesting that when my friend talked about her menopause my instant reaction was a sense of bereavement – and not many people think of it that way, but that was the first thought in my head. It's a form of bereavement.

LOW

(adj)

c.f. Low mood, a depression or time of sadness,
a lack of joy in one's life.

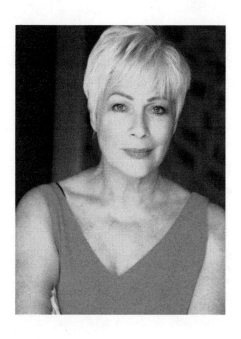

Denise Welch

Actor and mental health campaigner

"My bad times were outweighing the good and I was working in a fog of mild – therefore manageable – depression for most of the time."

Denise Welch, 62, is known for her roles in *Waterloo Road*, as a *Loose Women* regular and as a mental health campaigner. She has suffered from depression, which began postnatally, for the last thirty years of her life. She is the author of *The Unwelcome Visitor*, a memoir of her depression, and plays a key character in the menopause comedy, *Dun Breedin*. She has two sons and is married to the artist Lincoln Townley, who is fifteen years her junior.

~

My depression started thirty-one years ago when I had my first child. It began as postnatal depression. I'd never had any psychiatric or mental illness – not a day of it – before I had my child. So it was a complete shock, especially because I'd been the typical blooming woman in pregnancy. My hair was great, my skin was great, I felt great. I wasn't sick. I didn't even want the baby to come out, I enjoyed being pregnant so much.

So obviously I was floored, as were my whole family, when five days after having my son I was on the verge, apparently, of a puerperal psychosis. I can remember I was lucid most of the time, but it was a very scary time, and when people say to me, "Well, how long did you have postnatal depression for?", I say, "Well, thirty-one years." Because unfortunately with me it opened up a tendency to clinical depression that I live with to this day.

With the menopause it's hard to know when it has started or when you're in the middle of it. But all I remember is that ten or eleven years ago, when I was fifty-one and filming *Waterloo Road*, I found I'd got to the point where my bad times outweighed my good times. I had spent years in which a lot of self-medication went on, trying desperately to stop the pain of the depression. Also my depression in the main tends to be endogenous as opposed to reactive – so I have no control over when it comes on. So, by this time, I'd had twenty years of being poorly. It was just part of my life. For twenty years I had said to various rubbish psychiatrists I'd seen, "I'm sure that the origins of my illness are hormonal." And I'd had them say, "No, no, no."

But I'd think, Well, I had a baby. I produced a human being inside my body and after that happened, I was plunged into a suicidal depression, and you're telling me that could not possibly be hormonal?

So, at that point when I was filming *Waterloo Road*, I was aware of this feeling that the balance had shifted, my bad times were outweighing the good and I was working in a fog of mild – therefore manageable – depression for most of the time. It was not lifting in the same way that it had. It was only much later that I realised that this was probably the onset of menopause.

I remember, at a party, speaking to a friend of mine, Darren, and he told me that another actress friend of his had been to see this Professor Studd in London. He said, "She has depression very akin to how you talk about your depression."

The next day, while standing in the corridor of the school in which we filmed, I phoned Professor Studd's secretary and she said, "Can you come next week?"

I said, "Yes." She said, "Well, don't worry, we'll make you better." It was such a ridiculous thing but there was something about what she said that made me really want to believe in it, and I went down to see him. What Professor Studd found was that I was so low in oestrogen that he didn't know how I had survived. So he treated me for that. He also has massive success with the menopause, with women with depressive symptoms.

When Professor Studd prescribed the hormones they turned around how I felt. It was gel at the time – I have tablets now.

Carol Vorderman has been very open about her menopause and the depression she felt that she had never known before. Of course, I knew what depression felt like, so it wasn't new to me. I just knew it was becoming more persistent. I think for someone like her, who has never had any depression before, to suddenly have it when you think you have been there and got most T-shirts and then you're plunged into that, it's such a shock. Because I think a lot of people know the menopause is coming and are prepared for it – but they think they're just going to wake up with the sheets drenched at night.

They honestly think they will wake up and stick their head out the window and have to change their sheets in the middle of the night, and funnily enough that was one thing that didn't happen to me, that thing that everybody says they have – night sweating. Mine is just the all-day sweating.

I think my oestrogen levels had probably been low for a long time.

I remember going to see this specialist doctor and describing how my illness comes on. I said, "It can feel like a whoosh, where I'm flooded with something and it can be on me within thirty seconds." He said, "Oh, I think you have temporal lobe epilepsy." At that time I was so desperate to have temporal lobe epilepsy because I so wanted to have anything that they understood and could treat. I remember saying to him, "I have had a child [I'd had two by then] and I was a perfectly normal person until I had a child and I know that something like 80 per cent of women can suffer more serious things than the baby blues when they have a child. How would there not be a hormone imbalance when you have actually given birth to a human being?"

He said, "Oh no, no, no." He wasn't having any of the hormonal thing.

Then I went for the temporal lobe epilepsy test – and obviously I didn't have it.

When I was first poorly, thirty years ago, I went to a terrible GP who – bearing in mind I'd tried to throw myself out of a car – said to me, "I had five children, dear, and I just didn't have time to get depressed." That's what she said! Unbelievable. That's stayed with me ever since. If I didn't have the family I have, God knows what would have happened – they knew I was seriously ill and never doubted that this was something very serious.

All those years later, I said to John Studd, "Why has it taken me twenty years to get someone to consider that the origin of my illness is hormonal?" He said, "Well, because you've paid £500 to come to me. You think they want me to have that money?"

Yet the idea of a link between depression and hormones has always been around. Years before, thirty years ago, I'd met this woman called Katerina Dalton, and she's the woman who had coined the phrases premenstrual syndrome and postnatal depression, and she was treating women with postnatal depression and menopausal depression with progesterone. Then of course it transpired years later that it should have been oestrogen and not progesterone. But when I went to my GP, who I really liked, my one in the North East, he said to me, "I don't doubt, Denise, that this is something to do with hormones, but we just don't know. We just don't have the training in hormones."

So I was in the wilderness of not knowing what to do. I made the decision to start talking about this thirty years ago when I was a very lone voice in the wilderness. No one was talking about postnatal depression, depression and hormones. It was a very lonely time.

I don't think there's enough talk about all these different things that happen with menopause. I've noticed from the women I've spoken to over the years, a lot of people who have had postnatal depression, even those who don't live with it all the time like I do, go on to have a recurrence of depression during menopause.

We need so much more research into this. I've always said if men had postnatal depression and menopause there would be a clinic on every corner.

Also, we've always stereotyped women with postnatal depression or menopause or premenstrual syndrome in dramas or comedies.

"It's that time of the month."

"Oh, she's just had a baby, ignore her."

"Oh, it's the change."

They've always been the butt of the joke. I've got a big sense of humour. I'm not sensitive about everything. But I think there are other ways to use this, like we've done in *Dun Breedin*, a comedy that I worked on during lockdown in 2020. It presents menopause comedy where it's actually on our side, not from the male gaze.

I had no idea that talking about menopause, talking about incontinence, was taboo. But because I'm a very open person, because I do a show like *Loose Women*, I've always been open about things like that. I talk about wetting myself all the time. And I always find that if you talk about topics with humour it takes the edge off it. That's why Tena Lady asked me to get involved and I did a couple of posts for them and tried to incorporate humour. That's why *Dun Breedin* has been successful on YouTube and we hope to make a series about it, because we're all women at several different stages of menopause.

I'm sixty-two now. I have no idea if I'm through the menopause. Because what it has left me with is hyperhidrosis.

Basically, my body can't regulate hot temperatures. But my hormones that I'm on aren't stopping it. When I was having hot flushes, even if it was cold, I would still have a hot flush. Now if it's cold I'm cold, but if it's warm and everyone is just going, "Blimey it's warm," I am wet through. Wet through to the point that it looks like I've been in a swimming pool.

It's miserable and I've kind of learned to live with it, but it's why I spend as much of the summer in normal, non-lockdown life out of this country – because of the air-conditioning. I love nothing more than a British summer, but unfortunately hardly anywhere we go is air-conditioned – and it makes it miserable for me. Most of these red-carpet dos that we have to go to are in the summer and I really struggle with those. If I'm asked to present an award or, occasionally, accept an award, it's the first thing that comes to my mind and I've had to leave before because I've got myself so upset because I'm completely sweating through my dress.

I would like to see consideration. When people are hosting something or rehearsing something – not just in my industry, in any industry – where there is a cross-section of ages, then I wish they would think about the demographic of the people there and realise that a lot of people may be at this middle-age.

This sweating thing has changed my life and not for the good. I got help with the hormones, but unfortunately the HRT doesn't help with hyperhidrosis. When I spoke to my doctor about it, she said, "Denise, I could send you to a specialist, but I'll be perfectly honest it's one of those things we don't know why it happens." If it was just my palms or under my arms, where a lot of people sweat, I would probably have a bit of Botox or something semi-permanent, one of those things people do. But unfortunately, as I say to my friends, if I had Botox for my sweating, I wouldn't be able to move because it would be all over my body. I'd be walking like a Dalek. So I just have to suck it up. And think, To be honest if my head is okay, I'm okay. I can pretty much deal with other things if I'm feeling normal in my head.

I've had incontinence myself, all the time. I can't cough, sneeze, laugh, anything, without wetting myself. Some women are mortified by it, but I don't really care and I've been speaking to Tena about women who are far worse than me. Some women, if they cough or laugh, they proper wet themselves. Their wee flow happens as if they're having a proper wee. Mine doesn't happen like that. It's just a bit of wee comes out and I have to make sure I have a Tena Lady or a panty pad on, something like that. Mine is kind of deal-able with. But it has been embarrassing. I can laugh about it, but when it's happened and I've been out and not prepared and you're in the public eye, so there are eyes on you that may not be on other people... well, I've had to go home before.

We're made to feel like menopause is something that's our fault. Historically we were thrown on the scrap heap when menopause hit. Basically there was no more use for us, once we had done breeding, as it were.

I'm a huge HRT supporter... I think with me, because I've had such severe mental health problems over thirty years, you know when people say there's a risk of this and a risk of that, my mental health is too important to me, so I will gladly risk anything else.

For me, I am on HRT for my brain not for my sweating. Different people go on it for different reasons.

There is no one-size-fits-all for menopause.

I am in a really good phase of my life right now. I gave up drinking eight years ago with my husband, Lincoln. We both did and it's been the best thing we ever did. Not just for my life, but for the life of those people who love me and depend on me. I don't smoke anymore, I don't drink, I eat better, I try to stay moderately fit. I'm not obsessive about it. I'm in a much better place than I was in my fifties and my forties; a much better place, mentally and physically. And my Unwelcome Visitor, as my book is called, my depression, does not make his appearances as regularly. Last time he came was September 2019, a year ago. That's a long stint for me, touch wood. I haven't had an episode during lockdown, which has been great for me and also great for my husband.

> It's hard for me to say, for sure, whether that depression came because of the menopause. I think now, when I look back, that was the start of my menopause.

Lincoln and I actually met while I was going through the menopause. We both met in the madness as we call it – there was a lot going on in my life. My marriage was breaking down. I was self-medicating, which was making my depression worse, so then I'd drink more. I couldn't get off the treadmill. I met Lincoln and the press went crazy about it. We knew that the only thing ruining what would have been a lovely relationship was alcohol and we knew we were going to lose each other because the only time we argued was with alcohol, and so we gave it up and life is very different now.

We have talked about the menopause with each other. I'm very open with my husband about lots of things.

It's hard for me to say, for sure, whether that depression came because of the menopause. I think now, when I look back, that was the start of my menopause. My mum had a hysterectomy, so I never knew when the menopause would have started and I know there seems to be a correlation with when your mum started. I reckon I was about fifty-two. People say, do you think you're out of the menopause? I don't know. My sweating has continued. But is my sweating just something I've been left with? Or am I still in the midst of menopause? I don't really know. I don't know if there's a day when you think, Ooh, I'm not in the menopause anymore.

I'm certainly in a much better place than I was. I'm through the worst, for sure. And I won't give up on the HRT because it works for me. I think the onset of the menopause – which then resulted in my depression worsening and therefore seeking help and eventually finding help with the hormones – changed who I am. It forced me to get help. Otherwise something tragic could have happened because I was very, very poorly. But I wouldn't say I'm grateful for it. I've heard Stephen Fry say he wouldn't change being bipolar because it makes him who he is. I would change having depression, in a heartbeat. But it's something I've learned to live with.

When it comes to sex, I have a young husband, so that obviously puts a spring in my step. I don't know if menopause affected my libido. Depression does, without a shadow of a doubt. Depression completely kills the libido. My husband is very supportive of that, because usually my episodes don't last very long. But if I'm going back ten years ago, when I was depressed all the time, yes, menopause did kill my libido. My friend, who has vaginal dryness, says it killed her libido. They're totally frightened of having sex in case it hurts. I've not had that experience at all, but I think it's a really important topic to bring up.

The other thing is, I didn't realise that lots of women have problems with intimacy because of incontinence brought on by the menopause. And it's such a big thing, their embarrassment with that.

I try to bring a bit of humour into the bedroom, because again I think you can get through most things with humour. But, you know, I do think that the dialogue should open a bit more. I just didn't realise it was such a taboo. I didn't realise people didn't like talking about it.

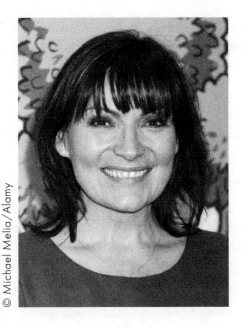

Lorraine Kelly

Television presenter

"That girl that gets buried because you become a wife or you become a mother or you're climbing your career ladder...she can come back. It's good to find her again."

Lorraine Kelly has been the queen of morning television for the last thirty-five years, presenting her show, *Lorraine*, since 2010. She is married and has one daughter. When, during her perimenopause, she began to feel flat, she decided the menopause was something that needed to be talked about on her show and created The M Word campaign. Her interviews with celebrities – including Carol Vorderman, Ulrika Jonsson, Meg Matthews – who revealed their struggles, have been key in helping break down taboos and getting the UK as a nation to talk about the menopause.

~

It was on a holiday in Cordoba, Spain, that it hit me that there was something wrong. I just felt flat. I think probably I'd ignored some signs – and maybe I was feeling a little bit more tired. But, you know, you're permanently tired if you work on breakfast telly. You get used to it. It becomes your natural state really. It's a little bit like being jet-lagged all the time. It's one of the very few drawbacks of the job – you just do feel tired. So if you feel a little bit like that, a bit exhausted, you put it down to the fact that, yeah, maybe you've had a couple of nights where you didn't sleep as well as you could and you were up early, at four a.m.

But this was almost like I went over a cliff. I think it had been building up – and I felt like I lost myself. It is awful when you lose yourself, you lose that sense of who you are. It's really scary and I can understand why a lot of women and a lot of GPs misdiagnose, saying that it's depression or anxiety. Yes, it is actually. But it's because you're going through this change – it's depression caused by the menopause and what you need to do is treat the menopause and not the depression. So it's difficult from that point of view. And it's not the GPs' fault necessarily. It's all about education and talking more.

I was really down. Joyless sums it up. I couldn't get any joy out of anything. I was on holiday in this beautiful place and it was gorgeous. You couldn't have had a more idyllic place. And I should have been really happy. Content, not happy – content is very overlooked and underrated. I should have been content but instead I was thinking, I don't understand why I don't feel anything. I just feel flat. It's like all the energy has been sucked out of my body.

It was like I could have got good news or bad news and it just wouldn't have registered really. It was a weird and horrible feeling and I never want to go back to that. Thank the lord it didn't last very long because I did manage to get it sorted. But I really feel for women who have to put up with that.

For me, it was a tiny, tiny experience of what it must be like to have some sort of mental illness – but obviously nowhere near as bad as someone who is clinically depressed. But you get a little bit of that sense of what it is.

It was Dr Hilary who diagnosed it. We are so lucky at work in having him there. In the morning there's always a queue for Dr Hilary, and especially now [during the Covid-19 pandemic] you can imagine everyone's very scared and wants reassurance and advice. Back then, I just said to him, "Do you know what, I'm just not feeling myself. I don't know what's going on." I talked to him and I told him the symptoms.

He said, "You're menopausal."

I thought, Oh right, great, good, we've got a label, we can do something about it.

You go away and you put your journalist hat on and you research it and find out what it's all about – and I found out everything I could and Dr Hilary was a great help. He put me on HRT. I put a patch on my bum and it changed my life.

That's what I did. I got a patch. I would say it probably took a month to fully work and it got gradually, gradually better. It wasn't like a switch. I know Carol Vorderman says when she put gel on her arm almost instantly she felt better, but for me it took a little bit longer. And it was like every day it got brighter. Every day I felt better, until I realised I was actually back to where I wanted to be and that was fantastic. But probably it wasn't that long. A couple of weeks to a month, I would say.

Then, of course, from that initially, things can change, as you know. Your levels can change, so it's not just that you get help and then you put a patch on your bottom and that's the end of it.

A couple of years ago, the symptoms started creeping up again. This time I realised what it was, and I went to Dr Louise Newson and got a blood test. She just said, look we have to up this dose and lower this one and you need a little bit more of this and a little bit less of this. And it's great. Because she's so good. What I would want is one of Louise's clinics in every city and every large town in this country. Because there are vast swathes of women out there who don't have access to the kind of help that Louise gives. I would love to clone her. There are still so many women out there who can't get help and that's just not fair.

I know HRT is not for everyone, but it worked for me and I still take it now.

Back in 2017, I felt we really needed to talk about this more on the show. Of course, it was a huge taboo and it was quite hard to get other people to talk about it, so in the end I said, "Well, I'll talk about it and Dr Hilary can interview me – we'll swap seats."

After that interview we had a massive response from viewers who wanted to know more and were desperate to talk about it, and Ulrika, Carol and Meg came on the show. We got loads of women – so, so many came forward. They just thought, This is great we're talking about this now. And it was wonderful that they spoke up because every single person who does that, through some ripple effect helps so many others.

When we did that show, I was astonished to discover the extent of people's anxiety. Some women in the public eye weren't really wanting to talk about it because they felt – wrongly I think, but sadly that's how they feel – that it would not be good for their careers because it was this sense that menopause equals old.

I never worried about that. But then, I think I'm quite unusual, and very lucky that I've got the nearest thing to a steady job that I can have in the world of TV, which still is a precarious career. But clearly being thought of as "old" is still a worry for a lot of actresses and female presenters.

So when I did that interview with Dr Hilary, it opened the floodgates. Its ripple effect got women talking about their experiences.

Honestly, we have never had such an outpouring and such a reaction from our viewers on anything we have ever done.

Some women were just saying, "Thank you, I thought I was going crazy." Or, "Thank you, I've now gone and got help." Or, "It's just good to know that's what it is because I thought my whole world was falling apart and couldn't understand what was happening to me." It's that sort of fear. As women we do tend when all of this is going on to keep soldiering on. We put ourselves on the bottom of the list. We always do.

I look upon the menopause very logically, as just another part of life. You become an adolescent and then you have periods and you go through all these different stages in your life.

I think there has to be a mind change; maybe we need a reset for people to stop being afraid, or thinking of it as negative. It's part of life.

We live a lot longer these days, thankfully, and we take care of ourselves a lot more. You look at some of the women who are around. I recently interviewed Twiggy, for instance. For the love of God, the woman is seventy. She's extraordinary. It's ridiculous. And you look at women in their seventies, eighties, and they're having a ball. And so they should be. This menopausal or postmenopausal time should be your time. It's your chance to do what you want to do. If you have had children, by and large, they're up and away, and it's your time to do what you want to.

I'm having adventures myself. I've gone on my wonderful trip to Antarctica, I've jumped in the Antarctic Ocean in my bikini. I've done all of these daft things because why not? I think you get to that stage which comes with hopefully getting older and becoming a bit wiser. I'm not sure. I still feel I'm waiting to grow up, waiting to find out what I want to be when I grow up.

That girl that gets buried because you become a wife or you

become a mother or you're climbing your career ladder, or you're doing whatever it is you are doing, she can come back. It's good to find her again. It's very freeing and very liberating. You can just do what you want, wear what you want, say what you want. I've certainly got far more feisty – although I'm not that keen on the word feisty. I've certainly got more opinionated and less worried about what people say and what people think.

There's nothing I wouldn't do. I've got so many things I want to do. I want to go to Mongolia, and I want to go to Greenland. We can't really travel right now but there will be a time post-Covid when we can do all these things. And we can push ourselves a wee bit, challenge ourselves and be out of our comfort zone.

There is also an obvious benefit of the menopause: the loss of periods. That was a joy. That was great. Not to have to deal with all that. I used to suffer quite badly with cramps and mood swings.

I didn't mourn their loss. I came to terms with the fact that I was only going to have one child some time ago. We would have loved more, but it just didn't work out. We didn't go down the road of IVF or anything like that, because I was very much of the view that if it will happen it will happen. I've been lucky enough to have one very happy, healthy child; I feel very blessed.

So, yes, while another child would have been fantastic, I still completely understand there are a lot of women who sort of grieve that the choice is taken away from them, that they don't have that choice anymore. For me that wasn't really a thing.

I remember talking to my mum about it and she said she kind of sailed through the menopause. She didn't really have any problems. Because of that I didn't have expectations that it was going to be a terrible thing. I was aware, though, that it was something that wasn't talked about. People just weren't comfortable talking about it.

And what needs to happen is that men need to be talking about it too. Because they also suffer. They don't understand what's going on. They're like, "What's happened to my partner or my wife, the person in my life?" You know what men can be like – "What have I done? How can I make this better?" They need to talk about it more and feel like they can broach the subject and it's not going to be treading on eggshells.

The menopause is considered to be a taboo, almost an insult, something to be ashamed of, which is absolutely ridiculous. I think that's why, when we broadcast the items that we did and still do, a few years ago, we got that overwhelming response.

People said it sparked a dialogue. When I was out shopping or in a café, women would literally come up and say, "Thank you."

> I actually like being an older woman. It's very freeing.

I did talk with Steve, my husband, about the menopause, and he was actually really relieved when Dr Hilary told me that was what it was, and to realise it wasn't anything horrific. It was simply a very natural process of growing older. It wasn't like a serious illness. I wasn't, God forbid, going down a deep well of depression. I've had a tiny small pinprick of what that's like, but for other people it's horrendous. I think he was just glad – it's something normal and every woman goes through it.

Of course I looked into the safety of HRT – there were a lot of quite scary headlines around a few years ago – but there have been studies done since and I feel I have made an informed choice, but it's all about what you choose to do.

I feel for me personally that the benefits outweigh any risk there might be. It can protect you against things like osteoporosis. It can help your mood and energy. And I can't be sitting there having hot sweats when I'm doing my job! Luckily, to be fair, that was not one of the symptoms I had and thank goodness. It must be bloody awful.

I've got such a good combination of hormone treatment now that I honestly don't think I've got any symptoms anymore. I'm always very aware that things could change, and indeed they might as I get older. But I can see me taking HRT forever. I don't have any reason right now to stop. Of course, some more studies might come out. There might even be a better form of HRT at some point.

I'm more aware of my body, I think, since this. I'm more aware of the changes and all the signals.

I would recognise feeling flat and beyond knackered. Especially right now.

I can differentiate between what is physical tiredness or mental tiredness from working or dealing with everything that's going on, and when it's beyond that and it's menopause.

We are all different. One woman's menopause is not going to be the same as anyone else's.

I actually like being an older woman. It's very freeing. I'm lucky in the sense that thanks to my mother, thanks to my grandmother, thanks to their genes, I've got more energy maybe than your average sixty-year-old and people are very kind and say that I don't look my age. I've had no Botox. I'm too scared. I've done too many items over the years of poor women ending up looking like something from Star Trek, ruining their lives. And I draw the line, personally, at cosmetic surgery.

So, I've not had anything done. It's just hit me. I'm not sitting there looking down on people. If it's for you that's great, do your research and make sure you get the right treatment and aftercare. But for me, no. I don't want to, I don't feel the need for it, and it's something I would be frightened of. I've got this thing – and I don't know if it's a Scottish thing or not – of "you don't go under the doctor unless there's something wrong with you". You don't go into an operating theatre unnecessarily. I have this thought of, Can you imagine if something went wrong? It would be awful, so no, I rule it out.

I'm very proud of my laughter lines.

I don't want to look like everyone else. Look at these TV shows of *Housewives of Wherever*, who all look the same because they've all got the same surgeon. To me, they look like they've been in a wind tunnel and I don't want that. But, you know what? If it makes them feel better, boosts their self-esteem and makes them feel more confident, great. Good for them.

I know that slight tweaks can help. People don't like something about their nose, they get it changed. But surgery to chase looking younger is not going to work.

You have to keep going back. I equate it with when you're in your house and you buy a new sofa and then you look at your living room and you're like, "Oh jeez, the curtains are looking a bit drab!" Or, "The carpet is not so nice!" That's the trouble; it's hard to know where to stop – and that's a real shame.

We mustn't be scared of the menopause. We mustn't be scared or feel there is something wrong because everything we're going through is natural. But obviously when it impacts on your life and when it's making you depressed and down and flat – you need to get help. Some people might sail through, some might have the worst sweats ever. I always say, "Don't suffer in silence. Get help. There is help out there. There is understanding."

And please don't just think, Oh it's the change. Oh it's women's troubles.

That drives me crazy that phrase – *women's troubles*.

That's why women suffered for so long with [vaginal] mesh implants. People were just saying, "Oh it's women's troubles." We don't say men's troubles. We don't say that when they're going through their midlife crises and all that malarkey. It's such a dismissive phrase. "Oh it's women's troubles, so the women can handle that."

We're beyond that these days, and we have to be. For me it's almost like the last taboo we've cracked – and thank the lord for that. I'm so glad we've got over feeling uncomfortable, or feeling it's not appropriate, and feeling ashamed. How can you possibly feel ashamed of something that's so natural?

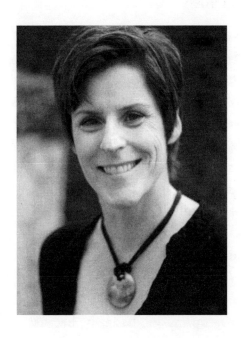

Helen FitzGerald

Author

"I remember the waves of anxiety. I thought, Oh, this is what mental illness is."

Helen FitzGerald is the author of many books, including *The Cry*, on which the BBC drama was based. She is a former social worker, married with two children. She tells here how menopause drove her to nervous breakdown, depression and leaving her job. Her crime novel *Worst Case Scenario* has, as its central character, a menopausal probation officer.

~

When the menopause happened to me, I thought I was having a nervous breakdown. Basically, one day I woke up – I was working in social work at the time as well as doing a book a year – and looked at the list of things to do that I write the night before, and burst into tears. It was just a list of all sorts of household jobs, kid-related things, paying bills and then at the bottom, write a thousand words

– and I remember seeing that, reading it, and then getting back into bed and bursting into tears from nowhere.

I remember the waves of anxiety. I thought, Oh, this is what mental illness is.

It went on for about a year of me just thinking, Okay, I've got really serious mental health problems – depression and anxiety. And certainly that is what I was experiencing.

It was a real tip over into something. One thing led to another led to another. Menopause is complicated like that. I got so tired and that made me incredibly anxious. The anxiety was the main thing for me really, but it was probably caused by the depression and the sort of exhaustion and collapse. I just couldn't get anything done, and because I'm such a busy person and I've always been so productive, I really found that difficult. I gave up my job basically, because I realised I wasn't coping.

I'd had some symptoms for a while. For a couple of years prob-ably I'd been having hot flushes and night sweats, and not sleeping well, mainly because of the sweating. I'd go to bed wearing the sexy outfit of a towel tucked under a T-shirt. My sister suggested it to me, saying, "This is how you do it. You put it under your arms and then you just tuck it out the top of the T-shirt and then you just put it between your legs and you'll stay dry all night!"

I would have been fifty or fifty-one in the run-up to that moment, and I was just getting upset, angry a lot. I remember once, somebody was taking ages getting a cup of coffee in the kitchen at work. And I actually imagined grabbing their head and smashing it against the tap. And then I thought, Oh God, I'm not in control. I haven't had a feeling like that, you know like a really impulsive rage, since I was a teenager probably.

It was pretty frightening in that job. In that job you really can't afford to not be on top of things.

At the time I was waiting to hear whether the television adaptation of *The Cry* was happening. It had been almost greenlit about a year earlier and then had just gone back to being on someone's desk because there was a change of head of drama. I'd decided to leave my work because, I thought, I'm bursting into tears all the time – and I can't do that.

But then I found I was actually able to leave because *The Cry* was greenlit. I rang my boss the next day, but I was going to anyway, or I was going to be on long-term sick and I didn't want to be on long-term sick.

Luckily, I also had a two-book deal. I wrote those books – *Worst Case Scenario* and *Ash Mountain* – and I don't know how I did it because I was pretty much depressed the whole time. The anxiety was really profound. There's a couch in the office and I would lie down there and think about a scene and then my husband, he's so lovely, would come up and say, "Right, get to your desk," and he'd sit there while I wrote it. I felt like my arms were made of lead. Just getting them to the keyboard was so hard. That's how I wrote those books – just one awful scene at a time.

It's really since I finished those books that I managed to get my life completely back together. I got into some bad habits. I feel like, because of the anxiety and depression that came with it, I stopped exercising as much as I once did. I really looked forward to a glass of wine in the evening and became, I think, dependent on that. It was the only thing that took the edge off the anxiety in the evening.

I've learned so much about myself. I've learned how to be happy. I'd never had CBT [cognitive behavioural therapy] or anything like that before, and actually, I wish I had when I was a lot younger. I started thinking about what triggers me and what are the day-to-day things that I need to be happy. I think through menopause I just really scratched everything and started again.

Initially, when the depression and anxiety hit, I just thought, Okay, there's a bit of a history of it in the family. I always felt that I was going at things too hard, working too hard and that I was probably going to crash at some point you know. I had an empty nest. The kids had just left home. All of those things I think come together for many women at that age. Elderly parents, too, becoming more frail. There are a lot of huge life stresses that happen at the same time as your hormones go bonkers.

I did go to my doctor to get the coil fitted because I was still bleeding extremely heavily. I now think, I was fifty, why did you give me one of them? At the time the GP did take blood, but my oestrogen level must have been okay on that day. The thing about those tests, they're not reliable.

It was my daughter, Anna, who said, "No, Mum, this isn't mental health problems, this is menopause." Thank God for Anna, because I had been getting so upset and staying in bed all the time, and she went to a friend's and said, "Oh, my God, my mum, what can I do?" They said, "What's going on?" And she said, "Well, she can't get out of bed and she's moody all the time." One of her friends said, "My mother didn't get out of bed for a year." Another said, "My mum has been crying all the time." So two of her friends said the same thing. And that's when Anna came home and said, "It's the menopause, Mum. You need to try HRT. You need to go back to the doctor."

So I went back with my husband. He said, "Even if the test comes back the same again, we still want HRT, you know."

I'm a bit of a conspiracy theorist about all this, because I don't really understand why it's so difficult. Is it just that they don't want to supply that amount of medication for that amount of time to half the population? Is it because we are just being viewed as whingey old women? I've got a theory about mother-in-law jokes; they're all really menopause jokes – they're being mean about women of a certain age.

So, in the end I got my HRT and it pretty much instantly took away most of the anxiety. You know, that terrible feeling of being at the top of a pirate-ship ride and not ever coming down. It immediately took that away – mostly. I still get it. I still have it sometimes, but I'm managing it and it definitely took most of the edge off it. It was instantaneous.

But I still had to tackle a lot of the behaviours that I'd developed. How much do I work? How do I say no to things? I feel like I've always been proving I can do everything. I can do it. I'll show you. I can have a job. I can be a writer. I can look after the kids. We can have a beautiful house. "You don't have to worry about that," I'd say. "I can do all that." But the truth is I can't. And I think menopause just shot me down and said, "Right, re-evaluate, what *can* you do?"

For me, it has been an opportunity to do that. I remember I had one good doctor before this, who said, "You need to stop caring for everybody." My sister had stayed here for several years; I'd moved over and lived with Mum for a couple of months while she was really ill. And it just, it was just nonstop stress, really. And this made me stop and say, "I'm sorry, I can't do that." That took a lot of practice.

I let some things go. I let the house go to such an extraordinary degree that I'm only just getting it back together – and I'm really into a nice house. It took me a long time of not doing anything for people to start doing them – to realise the bills hadn't been paid and stuff like that. You know, a little is my fault for sort of taking things on over the years and just thinking, I'll do it – it'll be quicker.

But my family are amazing. Anna, my daughter, was incredibly knowledgeable and supportive and Serge, my husband, is amazing, and Joe too. And it was hard for them. I'm sort of taking a while now to be normal again. I'm not having the moods that I had.

I wrote *Worst Case Scenario* just after I got the HRT, and its central character is a woman going through the menopause, with all that rage and no filter. I was still really fatigued, but I wouldn't have written it without the HRT. I started writing it basically as soon as I got the pill.

I don't miss my social work job. It was the right time. I've done it enough. I wasn't getting any better at it. But, although I don't miss it right now, I might next week. It sort of always pounces up on me – that feeling of oh I'm bored. I really miss that sort of excitement of that job; it's a really buzzy job. I miss meeting all those interesting people and the stories you get, but I don't have the temperament for it anymore.

I feel I probably did my bit towards the gender pay gap by leaving work and I probably shouldn't have left. I would probably still be there if I'd been able to take some time off and get the right help with the menopause, with HRT.

> When I watch *Love Island* and all those dating shows, I'm kind of bamboozled by what's going on.

The menopause has also changed my relationships. I think I have better relationships with men now. I was a big flirt. I mean, I was very happily married but I loved that buzz of being attractive when you go out. And I don't care about that at all anymore. When I watch *Love Island* and all those dating shows, I'm kind of bamboozled by what's going on. It's like a phase that I don't understand anymore. It must be so chemical, so hormonal. I'm not saying I don't feel sexual anymore. I do, but I feel like it's not the biggest thing.

My relationship with my husband has probably become stronger since – we really know each other better and, you know, I went through a lot of self-development. I think that's helped us too. He was just so helpful. And understanding! I'm really lucky to have him. We have a lot of fun together.

So far, I'm pretty lucky, ageing wise. I've got this sort of teenage boy's body and it's still a bit like that, which is great. I think being flat-chested at this age is a good thing. But yeah, I'm okay with it. I mean, obviously, I have aged. I look my age and everything, but I think I want to try and be the best fifty-three I can rather than trying to be thirty-three.

One thing I have noticed, and I remember a lot of women my age when I was younger saying this, is that I get interrupted. I am noticing getting interrupted *a lot*. But I'm wondering whether that's because I'm really snappy or just because if someone interrupts me, I want to kill them.

The menopause has changed me. I do feel different. I went to a counsellor and did CBT, which was incredibly helpful for me. And the discussions and issues we went through at home made us all know each other better. Relationships are different. I'm feeling more confident. I look after myself. I don't think I looked after myself at all really. And now ... I've never done my nails in my life, but you know through this lockdown, I've been doing my nails. A key thing I've learned is self-care. Looking back, I'm sort of mind boggled at how little self-care I ever did.

I think we need to talk and talk and talk about the menopause. I bring it up so many times, especially in front of men. I don't know if it's just to make them feel really awkward. And that's important – to start talking about it. I remember when people started talking about periods – my daughter has always been really open – how important that was. The more you talk, the less stigma there is. The more you hear something the less afraid people are of it.

Demystifying it is what we're doing.

STRONGER

(adj)

Physically and mentally more powerful;
competent and rich in resources.

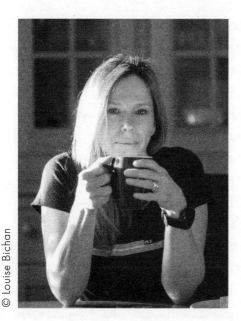

Erica Clarkson

Civil servant and ultra-runner

"We can choose not to be our mothers or our grandmothers. We can choose to be accepting of the menopause."

Erica Clarkson is Head of Rural and Island Communities for the Scottish Government. Living in Orkney, in her late forties she took up long-distance running, and in 2019 set the Guinness World Record for running an ultra-marathon distance on a 400-metre running track. She called that ultrathon the Meno Ultras, and ran it to draw attention to the menopause and raise money for Wellbeing of Women.

~

The menopause started at about forty-five for me – which actually is quite young, in terms of the kind of average age that menopause can hit women – and it peaked for me at around forty-seven to forty-eight, which is when I started to take my running a lot more seriously. So there's obviously a correlation there. I was a textbook case, apart from being a little early, of all the things that you'd expect to see – night sweats, rages, muscle aches and joint pains. And I had the most incredible anger, which was just not normal for me.

Until I really found my rhythm with running, it was poor Adam, my husband, who bore the brunt of my rage. I remember being in the kitchen one day and we were talking about something, I can't even remember what it was now, but it was obviously a little bit provocative because I was becoming increasingly riled. My eye caught a veggie knife in the cutlery tray of the dishwasher that I was loading at the time – and a rather disturbing thought flashed through my head! I didn't know whether it would be best to stab Adam to death in a bloody, frenzied attack, or whether I should have a crack at myself with that knife!

Deep in my heart, I knew I wasn't going to do either of those things, but I felt such anger – and that's not me. I have tendencies towards optimism, happiness and positivity. So that was really odd. I hated just about everyone – and I especially hated my work colleagues.

I think there's something about our generation where we have such a strong work ethic and such gratitude just for having a job. You know – it was like, I can't actually believe I have this awesome job, doing great things for people in rural and island communities. Seriously, I thought, well, I'm going to be found out for being an imposter, so I better work every hour God sends so that I can sustain this job. And also, in my wee family, we have something that's perhaps more common nowadays, but certainly was rare in previous generations, where I'm the breadwinner and my husband works part-time and is the main 'stay-at-home' parent.

You feel this enormous burden of responsibility to look after your family. And you do that by earning money to keep a roof over their heads. But with all these things going on, this rage towards my colleagues, I actually had to take time out from the workplace for the first time in my career. I had to take six weeks off, because I was just so lost. My mind was foggy, I couldn't think straight and I didn't trust myself not to bite the heads off my workmates every five minutes.

There wasn't a single trigger for all of this. It was more like this kind of perfect storm that I guess happens for many women, of having teenagers, feeling as though you've peaked perhaps in your career and having to sustain a crazy pace just to keep up with younger, brighter colleagues who are nipping at your heels. Oh, and not to mention having ageing and ailing parents. Some context, I have one child, my son Woody, who is fourteen. I've also got two older "bonus boys" because my husband was married before. They're pretty amazing.

My parents have both died now – and, actually, there's a sense of relief around that, too. At that time, I had a very sick father and some incredibly difficult sibling relationships – which, frankly, now I couldn't care less about. But at the time, because of menopause, it seemed like everything was just a disaster.

The other thing was, thinking about the workplace, I'd always been really sharp. But that changed. It's that foggy brain thing that comes with menopause. At the time I was the Chief Executive of the Judicial Appointments Board for Scotland, which is a pretty high-profile job in the justice world. The Board is responsible for making recommendations to Scottish Ministers for judicial appointments. It's a job with a huge responsibility for society. And, with a few exceptions, I was surrounded by the patriarchy, to all intents and purposes: white, older, middle-class, over-privileged men. I would go into these Board meetings, and I just lost my chutzpah. My stupefied brain let me down day after day after day. Unfortunately the balance in the judiciary still appears to be more in favour of men than women and I just felt incompetent to help change that. I felt like my brilliant team wanted me to be there for them, but I couldn't give them what they needed, and it became too much. Losing my sharpness and mental edge for me was one of the biggest – and more distressing – effects of menopause.

I had the immense lethargy that comes with menopause also, that kind of deep, never-ending bone tiredness. So yeah, the tiredness, the anxiety, the anger, the hatred of absolutely everything and everyone. And not to put too fine a point on it, I was getting pretty fat. I didn't like the way I looked. I know that's incredibly shallow to say. But, you know, just because I'm getting older doesn't mean I can't be concerned about how I'm presenting myself to the world. Yeah, that's where I was at. I feel like I'm underplaying it, underselling it; it was horrific.

For me, the weight had a big impact. I'm not a big woman. I'm very small, five foot two, and my racing weight is about eight stone. I'm naturally quite a light and petite person. But somehow in my early to mid-forties I crept up to over ten stone – for me that was way overweight. I carried it all around my arse and I didn't like it one iota. I hated it and there was absolutely no excuse for it. It is harder to lose weight as we get older and everyone you speak to will say that everything slows down and becomes more of a challenge. But I think perhaps what I was doing was using the ageing process as an excuse and using my quite full-on life and career as full-blown justification to reward myself with all the things I shouldn't have been eating, or to reward myself with sitting on the sofa at night and watching the telly and not doing something much kinder for my body.

Perimenopausal symptoms had started to happen before I hit forty-five. There was irregularity around my periods before then. They've always been a little bit hit or miss anyway – and super hard to track – but at around forty-six to forty-seven, they almost completely stopped. I don't think I've had one now for two years. Overall, there was a build-up of things for me. I think the best way to describe it is that I lost myself and my sense of who I was. I just didn't recognise myself anymore.

Looking back, there were other things too – like my hair was thinning out a bit as well. I also noticed that around my early to mid-forties I had all these mysterious aches and pains. Mostly, this manifested itself in my back, in my right shoulder and in my neck. I thought perhaps it was because I was driving and travelling, or I was working too much – you know – sat at a desk for hours at time.

I started running in my mid-forties, purely for health reasons. I was quite a good runner when I was younger. Well, I was light, like a little twig and I could zoom about the place and beat people in races. I was always in the athletics team at school and I was always on the track, bashing out interval training and trotting off to competitions and so on. I always felt that I could be good at it but I didn't have that encouragement that perhaps a lot of children who show promise might have from their parents, to really knuckle down and work hard. And then life took over as it does. You go off to college and then you have adulting stuff going on. You have to work really hard to create a home and to build your family and do all those things and I just lost my edge. I ran a little bit in early adulthood, but mostly to keep fit and never with any real consistency.

When I started running seriously again, I felt it gave me a little bit of agency over my body. I could control my limits and make time for myself. I have a wonderful coach, torturer-in-chief, who is called James Stewart – a GB and Scotland ultra-runner. He brings to me a straight aperture and focus and bucket loads of encouragement. I like the fact that the training gives me structure: consistency and a clear direction through thick and thin.

One of the things about running is it does release you from being the worker or the writer or the mum or the wife or whatever it is that you have to be most of the time. You can just go and be an athlete. And I loved that during the perimenopause and the tough menopause years, because it brings a bit of white noise to your life. You don't have to think about anything. It's not complicated. Running, perhaps less so in urban areas, but certainly running on an island is quite a lonely endeavour. And in a way that forces you to just "be" with yourself.

But the problem I found with the running was I was super-slow and my endurance was really off. But a lot of that was mindset as well. And I was really horrified by the fact that I was getting older. I was thinking, I'm old, so who am I kidding? I'm never going to be able to achieve anything as an athlete.

I was constantly looking for a "how to" guide for older athletes or for women who didn't want to become their mothers. I became almost obsessive about the research. And that's when I came across the charity Wellbeing of Women. Some of the articles and the research they published around HRT and menopause symptoms were the most useful reading that I could find. There were a couple of sports books where they lightly touched on older women trying to train and remain competitive through menopause. But they were talking about osteoporosis, slowing down or giving yourself more recovery time. All the things that just ring of old age – for me as an athlete at least.

I found that particularly in running and sports literature, the advice for menopausal women is very, very scant. Running and athletics is all about the young. And rightly so. They deserve that moment. They work really hard. But older athletes work hard too. We often have busier schedules and more on our plates, but we don't get recognised unless it's in that voyeuristic way of looking at a bunch of ninety-year-olds race each other around a running track, because people see it as kind of freaky . . . But it's amazing. Wouldn't you love to do that when you're ninety?

But in my mid-forties all that wasn't seeming possible. I knew I was in the perimenopause and needed to seek out some help. I have a GP here. His name is Huw and he's a wonderful man and an athlete himself. He's deeply interested in his patients and we're very lucky to have him on the island. I went to see him and I said, "I think I'm perimenopausal or even menopausal, because this shit is happening and it's real and it's not me." And he said, "You know what, I actually don't know what to do for you. I don't understand enough about it. But I want to – so that I can give you the care that you need."

He did prescribe me something early on – oral oestrogen, I think – but it was awful. I had headaches and felt pretty sick so I guess it was the wrong thing for my body.

So, we both agreed that we'd go away, we'd research it a little bit and I contacted Dr Louise Newson via email, maybe Instagram message actually. I sent her my story and asked her if she could advise how Huw and I could get my prescription right. And she said, "Don't worry. You know what, I'm going to speak directly to your GP. Give me his details and we'll have a conversation." And that's exactly what they did. They spoke about me and what I needed and Louise made some suggestion as to what to prescribe. And that was just the most amazing good fortune for me. But you know how many doctors, men doctors, would be so receptive? The thing about Huw is he had no ego about it.

Huw prescribed for me Evorel patches and Utrogestan tablets. I recall that I took them on Bonfire Night two years ago. I whacked the patch on my arse in the morning and took the tablet later on that evening. I remember we popped into Tesco on the island to get some marshmallows for the bonfire. I had a dizzy moment and I thought, Oh no. This is just not going to work. Thank you, Louise, thank you, Huw, but I can see this is just going to be a recurring problem. I felt nauseous. But literally within ten minutes it had passed. The nausea had gone completely and it was like someone had flicked a switch. Honestly, I can't express to you how quickly the changes came about for me – within a couple of days I was up and running. I appreciate that HRT doesn't work for everyone but I will champion it to my last breath.

After the first couple of days I was sleeping through the night. I felt my energy levels come flooding back in like someone had opened the gates and I was also becoming more articulate. I started to get more of a sense of peace and calm and I felt more confident and I think there were physical changes too. My skin got better – less dry and grey. My hair came back thicker and was growing more quickly. My nails were stronger too. But mostly for me, it was things like I could get out of bed again and feel like I had a little bit of energy. Things improved even further when I changed-up my diet and committed fully to being vegan. Once I had eliminated animal products from my diet – combined with the HRT and the increased focus on training – I felt better than I have ever felt in my life. That sounds preachy, right? I make no apology!

We've tweaked the numbers a little on the HRT over time, but I feel now that we've got it absolutely right. And that wonderful opportunity for Huw to have that conversation has allowed him to help other women on the island as well. He's actually become really interested in his menopausal patients. So, maybe the whole thing has been a little transformative for him too. My son Woody, coach James and my husband Adam are also pseudo menopause experts. You're welcome, boys.

I still suffer a little bit from insomnia, I can't lie. Sometimes it's muscle soreness from a long training session or a race. But some-times if I get a bit too relaxed with my HRT, the first thing to come back is the sleeplessness and the night sweats. I also allow myself to get impacted by work stress sometimes. And that's when I realise that I've got to get my shit back together and get back on top of taking care of this problem.

I can tell you absolutely, I will never come off HRT. I can't sell it hard enough. It transformed my life. Give me all the oestrogen and I'll bathe in it. The aches and pains that were a constant kind of niggle that I'd put down to working and to being overweight just went. The better I got, and the more into the HRT treatment I got, the more things started to click into place. I've upped my game even further with lots of lifestyle changes now and I'm pretty much pain free right now – and have been for quite a while – so I can talk about what I feel attributed to that.

I had experimented with changing my diet before. I took a lot of solace in food during the "dark perimeno years". I think I felt before that it was my God-given right to eat whatever I wanted, but I hated myself. I think again this is generational for us, that older woman can associate food with not necessarily good stuff. We think that we need to ration what we eat because otherwise we'll be fat and we can't be fat. Ever. So we deprive ourselves of things. I no longer do that. I enjoy food just as much as I ever did – it just takes a lot longer to bloody cook it now that we're a vegan household.

I run around three to five miles every morning before breakfast because I feel there's some benefit in doing a slightly depleted run – especially for endurance athletes like me. In races, I'm usually good up to about forty miles, but then my body starts to protest. I ran the West Highland Way race in 2019, which is ninety-six miles, and I was horribly slow because I was vomiting pretty much for the last fifty miles. So, I've introduced these depletion runs to my training so that I'm used to running on empty and I think that helps with kind of balancing my weight as well as it sets my metabolism up for the day.

It's not hard to do. I live on a windy island in the far north, so if the weather's bad, I tend to run on my treadmill – also handy because I can bolt to the loo if I need to. Then I usually have a second session in the day, which is either a really long run or it can be an interval of hills session or whatever Coach James asks of me. I'll also do some weights and mobility work at least five days out of seven – I have a great little gym set-up at home. I try to do my morning yoga flow Monday to Friday.

During the coronavirus pandemic my work has been off-the-scale intense. I lead the Rural and Island Communities Team for the Scottish Government. Obviously rural communities are really vulnerable to Covid-19. Many have an ageing population, variable supply chains and less-than-ideal access to medical services. So, to serve them well and to look after my team, I have to be extra disciplined. I usually get my pre-breakfast run done between six and seven a.m. and then sometimes I'm finally running at eight or nine at night just to try and fit everything in. I generally sleep a lot better than I did before, but the only times I notice I'm not sleeping so well is if I've not kept on top of changing my patch.

I'm lucky. I have a nice life. I don't have many worries – but you know I have a full-on job and a family to look after – so it's not all skipping along the beach and dipping my toes in the waves. But I do genuinely think without the HRT, my menopause would have been a whole lot shittier than it was.

The other thing I do is drink lots of water. We sweat a lot more as we get older. When I'm training I'm very, very, very sweaty. I only drink a wee cup of coffee before two p.m. in the day. I also take nutrients to supplement my diet. I take Vitamin D, B12 and magnesium. I also take omega 3 and an iron supplement every other day – partly because I run a long way every week and can get pretty tired.

One of the things that has worried me about menopause is getting osteoporosis. There's quite a mixed range of views in the science about whether running is really bad for your joints – or whether it's beneficial. I do have a bit of a monastic focus on my training and wellbeing, and I understand that not every woman can do this. I lift heavy weights, doing low reps most days. The reason I started doing that was because I was terrified of osteoporosis and falling down while out on a nice trail running and breaking a hip like a wee old lady. This is something Coach James and I are addressing in my training. I've become very tentative on downhill running. Something in my mind is saying, "You're going to break your hip. Just mince down this hill like a ninety-year-old woman and you'll be fine." We're working on this!

In the winter of 2019 I set the Guinness world record for the most consecutive days to run an ultra-marathon distance on a running track. I ran fifty kilometres a day for ten days in a row. We called it the Meno Ultras and yes – it was really, really hard. My body put up a bit of a fight towards the end, but I got the job done. One of the wonderful benefits of the challenge was that it brought people across the island together in such an incredible way – of course, it helped to bring menopause issues out into the open. All these farmers and fishermen and island men were coming to the track and saying, "So why are you doing this?" I'd say, "Well, you've heard of the menopause?" and we would have a conversation about it and it was just incredible. And wee kids were coming out to run with me too. Kids, seven to eleven years old, hearing about the menopause. We teach kids about periods at school, about childbirth, but menopause doesn't get talked about – perhaps because menopausal women are still perceived as being old, dried-up, has-beens, our careers are coming to their end and our lives are over. Well, I'm not having any of that nonsense.

Right now, I don't win a lot of races, because at the moment I'm in a category where I'm competing with forty-year-olds. But I'm about to go up an age category and I have an ambition to try and get on the podium a wee bit. I've got some bigger races lined up. My torturer-in-chief and I are thinking about another world record attempt, which is kind of a secret right now. I'm also thinking about chasing something called a FKT (fastest known time) here on a local trail. Setting those ambitions for ourselves is really important as we age.

I've never been elite and I'll never, ever be close to being elite. But this kind of attachment to my physical self and my physical abilities means that I don't see any reason why I can't strive to be the best fifty-year-old runner out there.

> If he has a question about running and health, he asks me – and I feel so proud of that. He believes that my opinion is worth listening to and I hope I'm setting a good example for him.

Why can't I do that? Yeah, I don't have the advantages of youth when it comes to recovery time and I lack speed in my legs. I don't have the daring of youth, but I still feel very strongly that women of our age and our stage in life can still have ambitions – physical ambitions around their sport. One of my inspirations has been Louise Minchin. Her book had an amazing impact on me. For me, looking at her and her life stage and how she tackled her sport and became, you know, really amazing, well – that's just fantastic, right?

The ageing process will slow us down as athletes anyway. That's just what happens and I accept that fully. We're never going to hit those heady speeds that we had when we were younger. But what we are better at doing as we get older – and this I think is mostly women

– is absolutely nailing the endurance side of our sport. Certainly, that's where I've found my strength.

And, actually, I kept wondering: Where's the literature around this? Where's the literature around menopause and competitive sport and physical wellbeing, and really understanding what was going on? It just doesn't exist.

Although there is a lot more in the media about the menopause now than there ever was, we've still got a lot of work to do. So our daughters don't have to experience the same barriers and difficulties and prejudices that we have. We have an opportunity at our age to show younger women that, actually, it's all right. Getting older is okay and we're supposed to be here. Our culture doesn't really celebrate age in the way that other cultures do.

Did I feel any loss over the end of my fertility? I often reflect on the fact that I've always had this vision in my head of a big kitchen table full of all my children – but that never happened and if I'm honest I do sometimes feel sad about that. But I have Woody, who is my whole life, and my two bonus boys. I guess I was busy doing other things and it's just the journey that I went on. I feel we were very lucky with my son. He's an incredible boy and he's very athletic. He's built like a whippet and he's fast. If he has a question about running and health, he asks me – and I feel so proud of that. He believes that my opinion is worth listening to and I hope I'm setting a good example for him.

My mother didn't talk to me about her menopause. She was an unusual woman. I had a good enough childhood. There was no hardship. I had everything I needed. My parents were middle-class, hard-working people, but there was absolutely no affection in my family. My mother was cold and unloving. I can understand why. She'd grown up on an island in a very patriarchal society with quite a lot of poverty. She was also blind, which can't have been easy for her. She had some quite interesting tendencies and could have a wee bit of a vicious streak. I have one really strong memory of being a late teen and being out of the house and coming back one day. My mum had for some reason been rooting through my drawers and found my contraceptive pills. As soon as I walked into the house, she threw them at me – hard – and accused me of being all kinds of horrible things. Also, although I was a competitive runner as a youngster, I don't remember my parents coming to watch me at a single event. That's odd, right?

I had a better, more loving relationship with my dad who died in the summer of 2019. I literally came off the trail of the West Highland Way race and had to dash down to Edinburgh and nurse him through his last weeks. It was very traumatic and it resulted in a huge family bust-up. Grief and death does weird things to families.

My mum died about seven years ago, so wasn't alive during this menopausal phase. But had she been, we wouldn't have talked about it. She would have been embarrassed and I would have been embarrassed. But my dad, on the other hand, knew exactly why I was running and what messages I wanted to get across about the menopause, and he would proudly talk about it with anyone who would listen: "My daughter is going to break a world record, and she's doing it because she wants people to talk about menopause."

My journey through the menopause has changed how I feel about myself. Yes – for sure. I still have some worries about getting old, and I still have the same paranoid moments about, "Who am I kidding? I'm a fifty-year-old woman – everyone's laughing at me." Or, "I can't wear that dress or those short running shorts." We all have those "have I got too much makeup on?" moments. Or I'll sometimes think that I'm running and running hard and that makes me a bit of a sad, old wannabe in the eyes of younger athletes. But, overall, it has definitely changed my perception for the better.

Again, I can't emphasise how much impact HRT has had on my life. I'll forever be indebted to Huw and Louise for doing what they did for me. We can choose not to do age badly. We can choose not to be our mothers or our grandmothers. We can choose to be accepting of the menopause. It's not about a denial. It's just about living with it in a different way from the one my mother would have.

Menopause is not for the faint-hearted if it hits you hard. But it doesn't need to be like that. I think we can see it as a new opportunity. You're not saddled with monthly periods anymore. You're not going to get knocked up if you start having lots of wonderful sex with lots of beautiful men if that's what you want to do. There are many opportunities, so let's get after them!

I strive to be the best version of my fifty-year-old self. It does take a lot of work – I'm not going to lie. You can choose to approach the menopause in a way that you will be defeated by it, or you can choose to see it as an opportunity to change your attitude and your principles. I know that takes a lot of work in itself, but that's kind of what I've done and I think that ageing has reminded me of the passing of time.

Again, it's a cliché but you just don't sweat the small stuff in the same way. I mean you DO sweat quite a lot – because menopause – but I certainly don't get as worked up about things as I used to do and I think that's a wonderful benefit of getting older.

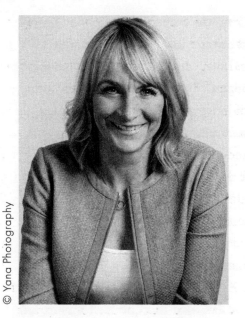

Louise Minchin

Television presenter

"I went to the doctor and they did the blood test and said, 'Yeah, you're definitely menopausal.' Actually they said 'perimenopausal' – but of course I didn't know what that was."

Louise Minchin, 51, is a journalist and television presenter who has hosted the BBC Breakfast show since 2012. In her mid-forties she started triathlon training and became a member of the Great Britain Age-Group Triathlon Team (45–49 age group). Her book, *Dare To Tri*, tells her journey from a BBC Christmas challenge of a bike race at the Manchester Velodrome to competing in the World Triathlon Championships in 2015.

~

I didn't realise the first signs of perimenopause until I'd been having them for about two years. I was talking with a friend of mine who was a GP about possibly having anxiety, and then I mentioned a few other things to her that had been going on – heart palpitations, night sweats and all sorts of things – and she said, "Well, do you think it might be menopause?"

I just thought, Are you silly? I'm way too young.

I was forty-four. I thought I'd be over fifty when it started to hit.

Then I went to the doctor and they did the blood test and said, "Yeah, you're definitely menopausal." Actually they said "peri-menopausal" – but of course I didn't know what that was.

Because of my huge ignorance about what the symptoms were, I had been suffering from related symptoms for quite a long time before I went to the doctor. I had thought they were night sweats and being hot – that's all. I had no idea there were any other symptoms, so had therefore been unable to connect what I was going through to the menopause at all.

I'd put the anxiety down to all sorts of things. We've all got stresses, haven't we, in our jobs? But it wasn't just anxiety. It was not feeling myself at all. I was genuinely worried that I had early onset Alzheimer's because I'd forget really important stuff. I'd forget words, forget I was doing something, put the car keys in the fridge. There were lots of things going on, but because I always thought the menopause was purely about physical symptoms, I had no idea it might be that. I just knew I really wasn't myself.

> "I was genuinely worried that I had early onset Alzheimer's because I'd forget really important stuff. I'd forget words, forget I was doing something, put the car keys in the fridge.

That feeling of not being yourself is really intangible and hard to describe. It's hard to put your finger on it. Not feeling yourself is very demoralising; it makes you lose confidence. There can be a kind of vicious circle in which you start to feel less and less confident.

People would say, "Oh, well, maybe you're a bit tired." For me there was always an explanation. It was always, "Oh, of course you're tired. You get up at three-forty in the morning." Or, "Of course you're tired, you've got two kids, two dogs, two ponies and the husband and a job." There was always a way to explain it away.

I felt I wasn't comfortable in my own skin anymore. I think my friends and family would have recognised there was something wrong. If I'd said to them that I just wasn't feeling myself, they would have said, "Yeah, you're right. You're not being like you used to be." Because I was always – and am again now – glass half full, always optimistic, always with a bounce in my step, always looking at what's next. But there was this negativity that crept in that wasn't my normal way to live. It wasn't the way my thoughts normally go.

We laugh about it now, my lovely nineteen-year-old daughter and I, but there were definitely times when she was going through hormonal changes, at about fourteen, and I was going through my changes and we met in this hormonal mess.

I would burst into tears. And I don't cry. It's not what I do. I would cry over ridiculous things, like *the* most ridiculous thing, like the fact I'd lost my car keys. There was no need to cry – they were safely stored in the fridge.

My daughter says I was half an hour late for an appointment because I was crying hysterically about something that really didn't matter at all.

But it didn't affect my work. Luckily. I have this weird thing where with work, thankfully, there's something about the pressure – and it is a pressurised job – that magically makes my brain fog go away. When I came back late yesterday, I was trying to have a conversation with one of my daughters that just didn't make any sense and I said, "I'm really sorry. I get up at three-forty in the morning. I don't know how my brain works when I am at work, but it does." It's like the red light comes on and something in the synapses makes it all okay.

I knew that lots of menopausal people can be diagnosed with depression. When I finally went to my doctor about it, I was having low moods as well. They offered me HRT pretty much straight away, and it turned things around massively. I know that people have their own issues with HRT and some people can't take HRT, but for me it was just fantastic. Within weeks it made a huge difference.

Though I went on HRT then, I had to come off it for medical reasons for a year or so. At the time I thought, Right, okay, let's see if I can manage this on my own. I'm going to manage it with exercise.

We know exercise is good for you and it's my absolute passion. It really helps! So much so I've decided my next book is going to be about the benefits of exercise.

It's really interesting because that was when I did a short film about my experience of the menopause on BBC Breakfast. I'd been asking them to do it for ages and, when they interviewed me, I was still really struggling. When I look back now, I feel I'm genuinely not that same person now. I describe my symptoms in the film, but I can't describe them as well anymore because I'm not in that same place.

Genuinely, I'm not such a shambles. I was really vulnerable then, so it was a brilliant place from which to do the interview because I was able, at that point, to vocalise something that many other people could see. Viewers were like, "Oh, that makes so much sense." But I can't vocalise it in the same way now because I feel so different.

HRT made a difference in so many ways. There are physical differences and then there are the rather less tangible, psychological ones. One difference between me on HRT and off HRT is that when I'm not on it, I can have up to four or five night sweats per night and, when I say that, I mean sweats like I have run a marathon in

Borneo. They are absolutely horrific. You have to get out of bed – some people I know have showers – so of course that really disrupts your sleep.

Another reason I wanted to see the doctor at some point was because I was having a really tight chest and heart palpitations, and then amazing aches. I would get out of bed in the morning and be aching, and then I'd explain it away as being all because I did a long run yesterday or I did this or that or whatever it was. There was always a reason why, but then you take the HRT and, suddenly, I could do loads of exercise and feel fine the next day.

My feet would ache, my bones would ache, I'd get cramps in the night. That's because if you're that sweaty, you're losing salts as well. There is all sorts going on that you don't realise. I'm also sleeping better because I'm taking progesterone and that apparently makes you sleep well. If I'm allowed to sleep, I'll go from ten o'clock at night till half nine in the morning.

The physical differences are amazing and then it's all those intangibles. There's the anxiety and, you know, we're living in anxious times and there are reasons now why anybody might be concerned for the future. I'm not saying I don't worry about stuff at all, but you don't want to be doing that worrying for no reason. And what I have found is those quite low moods I was having have ironed out as well. Even the forgetting of words; I still do that, but not nearly on the same level as before.

In that period before I went back on HRT, I think I was masking quite a lot of it by doing the triathlons. I'm a huge advocate for the power of exercise on both your body and your mind. I know it's my crutch, but that is what I've turned to during lockdown. If I go for a run I know I'm going to feel better; I genuinely do feel much better.

For me, when I wasn't on the HRT, I found that though exercise helped, it wasn't the cure all. It didn't solve everything and it certainly didn't take away those physical symptoms. Exercise was particularly a help when I was anxious and being naggy with the children. Even now my daughter will say, "Oh, Mummy, have you been for a run today?" I'll think, Okay that's a sign I need to get out.

With the exercise I have literally turned my lifestyle around. At university, I always was active and even when the kids were little, I exercised a couple of times a week. But for me now it genuinely is part of my lifestyle. It's what I do. It's what makes me get up in the morning. It is what makes me happy. The physical effects are sort of a by-product. I am stronger and I've definitely lost weight in the last four or five years. But that's all a happy by-product. What I really do it for is to calm my brain, to have a break, to get out, to be on my own, to not think. I think we're all so busy, particularly this time of our lives. We might have teenagers and might have parents we are looking after and we're probably holding down jobs as well. There's a lot going on for all of us.

When I run I don't think. For me, it's that hour a day every day where I'm not having to worry about anything or be anything. I'm not being Louise Minchin from the telly. I'm not being Louise Minchin the mum. I'm just being me. It's like a form of mindfulness. I'm not particularly into mindfulness, but that's what it is for me.

I'm fifty-one now and this whole exercise lifestyle thing started for me when I was about forty-five when we did a velodrome race as part of a BBC Christmas challenge. A few years later I was competing in the GB team in the World Triathlon championship, and then writing a book about it, *Dare To Tri*.

I've done some crazy stuff since. I think part of it is the risk-taking. I did a triathlon on Patagonia and it's called an Xtri, an extreme triathlon. You jump off a ferry in the dark, in the middle of a glacial fjord and you have to swim 3.8 kilometres and that genuinely is really heart-stopping. I was one of the last to jump in, but there's something about doing something really silly which is just so exhilarating. I hadn't done anything like that for years, if ever really.

There has been a shift in my approach to life during this menopause period. When I was a teenager I was really adventurous. Then you go through this period where you're holding down a job and you've got kids – and I'm really health and safety conscious with them, really risk averse with them – but I'm coming back to the point in my life where I'm going, "Yeah, let's go and do some crazy stuff." With that Patagonian Xtri, it's not just the jump off the ferry, it's the 180 kilometres on your bike, followed by a marathon. These are not small things to take on, but they're so empowering to do, to be a tiny part in this huge thing. It was so stunning. That's what I love about the outdoors – that you feel very small in this incredible world and it's really life-affirming.

I think I've returned to myself – but myself as a 25-year-old. I've returned all the way back, which is sort of brilliant. And this is an unexpected journey for me. If you had told me five or six years ago that I would be doing these things, I would have been like, "Don't be silly. Firstly they're not possible. Secondly they're not possible for me. I haven't got that kind of get up and go."

I want to make exercise a thing we all do, because it makes us feel great. For everyone to realise that it *is* for them.

There is an extreme triathlon in Norway called the Norseman, which is apparently the hardest triathlon in the world, and when I did it, people saw it on the telly. And now women have been and done that race because they saw me do it. My thing is to go and do stuff that looks crazy for someone who sits on the sofa and who is middle-aged. I like to make people think, Ah, maybe I *can* do something a little bit wild. Also that there will be another big adventure out there – I want people to know that.

To go back to confidence, I feel much more confident because I don't care so much. I don't sweat the small things. I'm prepared to stand up for myself a bit more than I probably would have done beforehand. In some ways it's my superpower.

I think we get to a certain age and don't care about things so much. I don't know if it's because I'm menopausal, but I certainly feel much more confident about standing up for myself and standing up for other people as well.

The other thing about the menopause symptoms is that before I did the film with BBC Breakfast I had no idea how many symptoms there were. Absolutely none. Experts say there are thirty-four. I would use those as a checklist and play menopause bingo with my friends. I'd say, "Right, here's the list. How many have you got?" When I was at my worst I was up to twenty-five or twenty-six.

That BBC Breakfast film was really amazing in that so many people watched it and for men and women it was like a light bulb going off. It was saying, "This is a real thing and there's help out there." What I was so struck by was the love and the generosity of women's partners going, "Now I understand. It's going to be okay."

I'm really positive about things now. During this lockdown, I've been feeling really well – I'm eating well and HRT is really working at the moment which is great. But the thing I'm sad about is that two-year period when I didn't know what was going on and when I felt really anxious and all the rest, when I wasn't myself . . . that I went through that and put my family through difficult times which I wouldn't have done if I'd known where to get help beforehand.

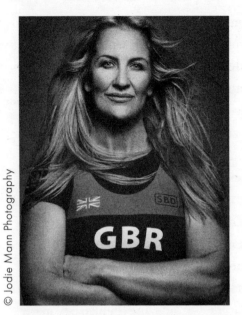

Melissa Wall

Powerlifter

"I was determined this phase in my life would be a time not of hardship but of opportunity."

Melissa Wall, 54, is an international powerlifter, who is currently the British champion in her class, a European and World Medallist and represents Great Britain in competitions around the globe. At forty-seven, not long after the hot flushes and night sweats started, with her kids grown up and an empty nest, she started powerlifting. Having watched her grandmother and mother struggle through their menopause, she was determined this phase in life would be a time not of hardship but of opportunity.

~

It was when I was in my mid-forties that my periods started getting a bit all over the place and the fatigue started to kick in. I just felt like everything seemed to be a little bit harder to do. Then after a while my periods got super heavy and they lasted a week to ten days and I was having to use both tampons and towels to try and protect myself. I thought, This is a bit rubbish. I've not been used to this.

That was followed swiftly by the sweats, the creeping feeling where it comes from your chest and up your neck and it feels almost like an anxiety attack. It started to click that this was all linked. Then came the horrific night sweats where I was literally soaked. I would wake up drenched with a little river running down my chest. I actually wrecked our mattress because there was this sweat patch where my body was.

I do remember having mood swings that were pretty bad but I don't feel they were any worse than PMT mood swings. I had hot flushes. I remember I would be sitting in board meetings and I would sit near the door so I could go out to the toilet and compose myself to come back in. There was that kind of rush of increased anxiety at the same time. I still occasionally get that, but I recognise it now for what it is and I know it passes really quickly.

In the middle of all this, at about forty-seven, I started powerlifting. My husband was a serving officer in the army and he was away a lot. The kids had grown up and left home. I was working full-time and I was into exercise. It was like a perfect storm. I had that "me-time", which my mum and my granny, that generation, didn't have, and it was something I'd always thought I would do – take that time, use it. Because it was something they never had the luxury of at that stage in their lives.

I always remember my granny's symptoms of menopause. She'd had a daughter Rita, my aunt, who'd contracted measles as a child and was left severely disabled. My granny brought her home and was determined to keep her there, and did so even well into her seventies. She would not allow her to go into residential care so Granny was a really remarkable woman and I always remember her having to lift and lay down this adult woman, my aunt, and wash, feed and care for her. She would have to stop quite a lot and she would say, "Oh, I'm having a hot flush."

As a kid, I didn't know what she was talking about. I would see her clawing at her neck and I knew it really upset her, but I didn't understand why. Her life was hard – though to her she was just doing what she could for her daughter.

Then, with my mum, she was running a business, as well as babysitting our children – because my sister and I were back at work – when she had her menopause. That was pretty rubbish as well. Again, she would say the same thing, "I'm having a hot flush," but I don't think until you start experiencing it yourself, you pay much attention to it.

I feel like their lives were very difficult at that age and mine has been so much easier. I've had the luxury of being in my late forties and being able to make a choice and do something for me as a sport. Powerlifting came into my life on the back of a New Year's resolution to learn something and make use of my time while my husband was in Afghanistan. My husband had challenged me to learn to do a pull-up in the gym. I knew it was a really difficult thing to achieve and that was when I sought out my first coach, who was a powerlifting coach, and I said, "I really want to learn how to do this while my husband is away, can you teach me? I'll pay you for a few sessions." But, of course, that quickly spiralled into the powerlifting.

Powerlifting and competing led me to completely change my career; after seventeen years of working for the government in a desk-based job, to studying to be a personal trainer and coach. The menopause has been positive for me in lots of ways, because you absolutely reassess everything. It's making the most of what you've got. Again, I had the luxury of a husband who supported me in doing that, in making that decision. Not everyone has that luxury.

I don't think powerlifting comes easily to me. Apparently, I'm the wrong shape for it, because I'm very tall and long-limbed, so I've had to work a little bit harder than some women. But I broke Scottish records in the deadlift at my first two competitions – that was a movement pattern that comes naturally to me because it works well for my levers. It's like anything – if you want to be good at something you have to work hard at it.

The training is hard. It's quite an extreme sport at any age. That mental toughness to go and put yourself out there for your country is super important. I compete in the Masters, so I'm competing with women in the same age and weight category, who are going through the same things as me, so it kind of levels out the playing field. My competitors will be menopausal as well. There's a terrific camaraderie in the powerlifting community amongst the women.

> Physical strength increases mental strength, so I can see how when you don't have control of things in your life due to the menopause, you want to take some of that control back.

My feelings about my body have changed a lot. Before I was powerlifting, when I was purely running, I was not eating very well. I was very light. I thought carbs were demons until I educated myself. Then when I got into powerlifting my whole mindset changed because all I cared about was being stronger – whereas before I really did only care about being skinny. My coach encouraged me to put a bit of weight on and to eat correctly and go up weight classes – I've actually put on ten kilos since I started.

And I'm loving it – and it's not all muscle, there's a little extra body fat too, but I actually like my size now. I think it suits my age. I can honestly say I feel in my best shape ever. That's really weird because it's a number on the scale which would have terrified me before. But I have had to eat to do that. I've had to eat quite a bit to do that. Donuts and cake; yes, bring it on!

I think we can fall into that trap with the menopause of feeling this is something that's happening to me that I can't control. But there are variables that we can control. We can't just give in to it. We're working later in life and we have to be fitter and stronger. Our families are probably relying on us a bit longer, and we're living longer.

I have taken HRT from quite early on. If I hadn't been competing in a sport I might not have done it so quickly. I just knew when the effects were starting to take place that they were really going to affect my training. When I weighed it up and spoke to my GP, I just thought, This is a no-brainer. Why would I suffer? I want to be doing good things. I want to be having fun at this stage of my life and if it means taking HRT and increasing my risk slightly then I'll take it. That was my choice.

It's interesting and exciting that so many women are getting into weight-training and powerlifting midlife. Physical strength increases mental strength, so I can see how when you don't have control of things in your life due to the menopause, you want to take some of that control back. Plus, the benefits in terms of osteoporosis are not a myth. I've read so many studies about it; just increasing resistance training by a marginal amount, and it doesn't matter how late you start, you're going to feel the benefits further down the line.

Longevity is super important to me. I want to be able to get off the floor if I have a fall, or to stand up quickly off a seat – that's just so important because it's not something I've seen in my mum or my granny. My mum is not a very fit lady for her age and to me she's relatively young. She's seventy-six, and she struggles to walk properly due to underlying conditions. So I've learned that, physically, it's even more important to me to be stronger than that when I get to that stage.

I watched the struggle of my mum and granny at my age, and though I've always admired them, I felt sorry for them. Our expectations at this generation have changed. We expect more, we demand more.

SPARK

(noun)

A small fiery particle thrown from a fire, which ignites other materials; c.f. sparky, lively and high-spirited.

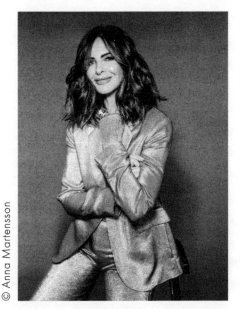

© Anna Martensson

Trinny Woodall

Television presenter and entrepreneur

"What can I do now that gives me energy, that looks after my body, that looks after my mind, so I can be totally in control of my body as long as I want to be? That's where I'm at."

Trinny Woodall, 56, came to fame as one half of Trinny and Susannah, the *What Not To Wear* team. In her thirties, diagnosed with infertility, she had numerous rounds of IVF before giving birth to her daughter, Lyla. In her mid-forties, when she was investigating her fertility again, she discovered she was already deep into the menopause. By the time she hit her early fifties, she had reinvented herself as an entrepreneur, launching the makeup brand, Trinny London.

~

I think I have more energy now, in my fifties, than I've ever had in my life.

I probably was about forty-five when I started experiencing the menopause. I'd always been told that you usually started menopause when your mother did. But my mother never acknowledged menopause because she was from a different era. Retrospectively, when I look back, I see there was a time when she was a bit short tempered perhaps, when she was fifty-five and I was about eighteen, and that's when we had a very tough relationship. I put two and two together and thought that was probably the menopause.

So I suppose I had at the back of my mind the notion that I would go into menopause around fifty-five too. But, in fact, it turned out that in my forties I went to have my levels checked and everything was already gone. I was already there.

I straight away went to see my doctor, and they put me on basic HRT without doing any blood work. It made no difference. So I went to see the bioidentical hormone specialist Marion Gluck, and I remember I spent £800 on tests and I thought, God, what a rip-off. But what it came back with was that I had no oestrogen, no progesterone. I was literally zero on all of them. Marion took forever to try and get me up to levels, using lozenges and bioidentical hormones, and it kind of worked.

What's interesting is that many women, when they go through menopause, happen to be going through things in their life anyway. You wonder, does one galvanise the other? It's a chicken and egg moment. At the very beginning of the hormonal changes, I was separating from my husband, the father of my daughter. Big life-changing decisions.

I see myself as very blessed to have Lyla, because I had unexpected infertility. I went and did nine IVFs and I lost a few babies, but then I had her. Then after, when I thought I'd try and have another child, I did another six rounds. By this stage I was forty-eight, and I was dealing with it.

After separating from my husband, my career was also changing, everything was happening, and at the same time, I just thought I want to go and talk to somebody for help. I'd read Suzanne Somers' book on the menopause, *I'm Too Young For This!*, which was a really amazing book for the time because there was nobody else writing about it with alternative solutions. I remember thinking, Oh my God, she takes twenty-eight supplements a day. Is that just crackers? Is that really doing anything? But I read that book, and it had an impact on me.

Then, a few years later, I kept hearing about this woman, Dr Erika Schwartz. She was in New York; she's a doctor, an endocrinologist and hormone specialist. So I went to see her. And it was like a revelation. First of all, the testing they did in America was so very different. I spent the morning there. It cost me a fortune. I was earning quite good money, but it was $6,000, and it was just insane. I did all these tests; they tested from my skin to my brain to my memory to my, you know, my puff to my hormone levels to my DHA levels ... Every single level, my pituitary, everything. And then Erika came back and she makes a decision based on all those things. So then I took all the bioidentical creams, and they just immediately began to work. And I took a lot of magnesium which I'd never had in my life, a lot of Vitamin D since my mother had had osteoporosis.

I just began to feel better. I remember previously my energy had gone. I'd even wanted to have sleeps in the afternoon. I'd go through months working really hard filming and then I'd have a couple of months off and during them my body was so exhausted that I'd just take a kip from two to four, which is very unlike me because usually I would do an eight till eight day. But I noticed after that set of treatments my energy came back. And I think, in terms of a successful plan for going through menopause, if you get your energy back, you know you're on the right path.

Then I got to know Erika, and now I do a lot of Instagram Lives with her as well. Erika is interesting. She is in her late sixties and she has some very strong opinions on things which people might just cringe at. She talks a lot about women wanting to look younger. She also believes very much in your sex life. Erika is really passionate on sex and says things like, "If you're not having sex with your husband, he's having sex with somebody else."

So when she said that on a Live, my community of Instagram women objected. Is sex essential to your life as a woman? Many women would say it's not – that they've got their girlfriends and they get love from that and they don't need that level of intimacy. But one thing I have noticed is that any woman who has gone through menopause who has a really sexy sex life has that energy. I'm not saying she has the sex life because she has energy. I just think you never find a woman who has a healthy sex life who doesn't have energy.

After that time with Erika, where she put me back on track, I was really diligent for about three or four years. You get to a stage in menopause where you've got over the worst symptoms, and I think what happens then is you kind of take your foot off the brake – or your foot off the pedal about what you're doing. I thought, Well, her products are expensive; I won't take anything.

I then found myself a little bit lacking in energy but not enough that I was going to make a trip to New York or talk to her again. So instead I spoke to Shabir Daya at Victoria Health, because we talk a lot about the menopause, and he has a kind of different route. His is to take supplements like magnolia rhodiola, sage complex, cherry night powder. It was a very different, very nice journey.

So I did that for a bit, and now I sort of pick up what I feel my body needs. I've learned quite a lot. I do know now that I want to stick with the bioidentical path because, as I go down the path of life, I want to support my creaking bones. I need the help of some form of HRT to do that. Like, let me double my dose of magnolia rhodiola... That gives you an instant boost.

I also take a lot of really good supplements. Erika can be black and white about it; she can say, you know, as your body feels there's no hormones there, it will slowly get ready for death.

A lot of people take affront to that. But I think if you take away the word "ageing" and you put in the word "energy", then it sounds a bit different. A lot of people might say, "Can't you just grow old gracefully?" Or, "Why do you need to do that?"

> But, for me, I do it because I want to be eighty and climb a f**king mountain.

But, for me, I do it because I want to be eighty and climb a f**king mountain. I don't want to be eighty and be my mum with Alzheimer's in an old people's home. I don't want to be that eighty. So how am I not going to become that eighty?

What can I do now that gives me energy, that looks after my body, that looks after my mind, so I can be totally in control of my body as long as I want to be? That's where I'm at.

I really do think I have more energy now than I've ever had in my life. And that's to do with a few things. It's to do with the fact that when you turn fifty, you assess your life. You have a checkbox inside your head which you feel defines you by the most obvious definitions, which is, have I been a mother, have I had a nice relationship, do I feel comfortable in my work or whatever gives me the pleasure during the day and gives me my life force, you know? Do I own my own home? There are ways we think this is a measure of our success.

When I reached fifty, for those first couple of years it was a time in which my career – my old career – was totally dead, and I was in the middle of starting a start-up. My daughter's father had died. There was a lot happening around me, which were very tough things to go through, and it was the time when I really needed to have the energy to deal with those things. It was the time when friends around me were saying, "Just get a job and be able to pay your mortgage."

I was in a house that was way too expensive for me and all that sort of stuff. But there was also the thought inside my head that if I don't do it now I'll never do it. So then I realised I had to sell my house. I had to pay tax bills. I had to sell lots of things I owned, so I could continue to fund that start-up business until I reached a stage of getting to institutional investment.

That took a lot of energy. I've said in interviews that when I turned fifty I stopped caring what people think, but it is actually more true to say that when I turned fifty-two I actually stopped caring – because all these things happened around fifty-one, and they were things I had to deal with.

For me, one key thing about Trinny London is that I'm not just building a makeup product people can buy. It's more like – how can I empower women and what can I give them to make them feel empowered?

Yesterday, for the first time in about three years, I looked in the mirror really close up because I was looking at something to do with a new product. I was in the magnifying mirror for about ten minutes. Lyla, when we do Instagram Lives, says to me, "Mummy, you've got these kind of trenches in your face." But because I'm fifty-six and I wear glasses I don't see them. But I saw them yesterday.

My partner Charles said to me recently, "Why don't you get one contact lens instead of glasses?" Because that's what he has done. He's had one contact lens done and got used to it.

I said, "Well, I would fall over because I'll lose my balance." But I also thought, I see my face as a twenty-year-old every day and I don't want to lose that. There's a reason our sight gets slightly worse – what you see is then how you feel about yourself. If I look and my face feels fresh, I then have tremendous energy. If I look and I feel I've had so much sugar and coffee and not enough water that I look drained, then I feel more drained.

Our looks are an indicator of our health. I can look at women and know a little bit about what they're doing – not just their skincare routines. And there's certain women who always had great skin, and then they get to their fifties, like Susannah, and they're saying, "I really need to get an eye cream."

I'm more fully myself on screen now. The thing about *What Not To Wear* is that we were very edited, so there was a sense from the team of what Susannah should be to women and what I should be to women. We were this yin and yang. More recently, after I started doing Lives, there was no one editing me, and that meant that what is on the screen is really, truly one hundred per cent, everything that I am in my life. It's allowed me to let those things come to the surface again. It gives me joy that I can make people laugh, even if it's inadvertently. I never thought I was funny, but the humour is just how I am and the eccentricity of what I am. But if it gives me joy, I don't care if people are laughing at me or with me or something in between. It makes me happy that I can make people laugh. It makes me happy that people can be inspired to do something.

One thing I've really learned is not to live in your past. That doesn't mean excluding every feeling from your past and keeping it shut up and becoming very, you know, full of undealt-with emotion. But what it means is you don't let decisions in the past control how you deal with the future.

Linked with that energy and being in the best place I feel I've been in my life is that I love myself. We can take a long time to get to a place where we love ourselves. I spent many years of my twenties thinking I wasn't good enough for what I was doing. I spent my thirties establishing who I was in a career. I spent my forties learning how to be a mother and I'm spending my fifties growing into myself. So I've grown into the woman I want to be and who I respect and admire, and I will give it my all.

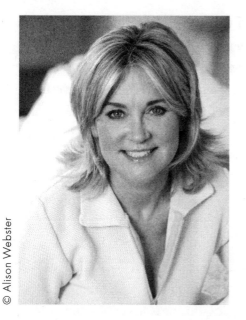

Anthea Turner

Television presenter

"But it's up to you. It's your mind. Youth isn't in a pot of cream. Youth is in your mind. Youth is about widening your horizons."

Anthea Turner is a much-loved face from UK television, who first hit our screens on *Top of the Pops* and *Blue Peter*, and later presented GMTV and *Wish You Were Here*. In her early forties, while married to Grant Bovey, she went through IVF which was unsuccessful. She is author of *How to Survive Divorce*.

~

The menopause brought with it a whole range of feelings; one of the most important is you're saying goodbye to your youth. For reasons that, to this day, I'll never understand, I never managed to produce a baby, but with the onset of the menopause – and even though my life had moved on from that loss psychologically – the curtain comes down and you'll never return to that stage.

I do think in the last six years we have begun talking about the menopause more. I began going through it when I was fifty-two, in 2012, and at that point I knew very little about it – in fact nothing, apart from the fact that your periods went all haywire and you had a few hot sweats. The way people talked about it when I was younger was all a little bit Les Dawson in his role of Ada Shufflebotham, mouthing the words "the change". Even my mum brushed it off as nothing, but I remember her being unlike herself for quite some time.

A friend of mine always says life makes more sense backwards and, when I think backwards now, I realise there was a time when my mum would have been absolutely in the age bracket, where she was difficult and she would cry and tell us off when I thought we didn't deserve that. I remember her having a go at my dad and driving off – which wasn't usually my mum. So now, thinking back, I realise that of course, she was going through all of this change, but her generation didn't talk about it. My mum maintains she had one hot flush and it was over. I don't believe that at all.

The only reason I had any conversations really about the menopause before its arrival was because I was very late to the party in terms of wanting to have a baby. People started saying, "You have to hurry up, because otherwise you know you're going to hit the menopause."

When I was thirty-eight years old, my now ex-husband and I began our relationship and my maternal instinct kicked in. I know some people grow up wanting a baby, but that wasn't me. I thought it just happens, which is another thing nobody told me – it doesn't always just happen.

In 1999, I started trying to get pregnant but things weren't happening naturally, and a gynaecologist said, "Look, you haven't got time on your side and if I was you, I wouldn't mess around. I would go straight for IVF. You can't wait – your body clock is ticking fast."

That was probably the first time I started to really have proper conversations about my "Down Belows". No one mentioned the menopause then; nobody ever said the word. It was more couched in terms of "before you get too old" or "before your eggs run out".

And even when they did speak about it, nobody ever said anything about what happens emotionally with the menopause – it was purely the bodily system. No one ever said what it does to your hair, your skin, your life, your sex life – none of that. None of those conversations ever took place.

Nobody sits you down and tells you about the menopause.

> No one ever said what it does to your hair, your skin, your life, your sex life – none of that. None of those conversations ever took place.

But once the perimenopause happened, I think I was embarrassed because this is the first admission of age and it doesn't necessarily show on your face at this point; this is your internal structure taking over and saying, "Girl, I know your eggs weren't much good in the first place but now your reproductive opportunities are well and truly over and all those endometriosis stomach cramps, piles of painkillers and hundreds of tampons were a total mitigating waste of time."

When I did start to have more dramatic changes, the biggest thing I noticed was that I just didn't feel right. I'm historically a fit healthy human with loads of energy and this was a shock for me. I couldn't put my finger on it. I wasn't feeling very well, not sexy. I was looking in the mirror feeling dull and sweaty. I couldn't quite get my head around what the problem was. You just don't feel the same – it's the weirdest, weirdest thing. And it's a shock and you're embarrassed; you don't really want to talk about it.

I did try and talk to my husband about it, but he wasn't interested. I even wrote him this letter, which I found when I moved. Going back to the phrase "life makes sense backwards", he had taken up with a 24-year-old so of course he wasn't interested in his sweaty dull wife's problems.

I said in the letter to Grant, "I just want you to know what's happening." I gave him a little bit of information on the menopause which I'd found. I said this is what's happening to my body and I'm so sorry, but I'm just not being myself.

I felt that I was being miserable. I was struggling to be as active as I would normally be. Finally I went to see this lovely doctor at my local NHS practice. I sat down with her and burst into tears and said, "I really don't know what's the matter and I've been here before and one of the other doctors gave me some tranquillisers but I really don't want to take them." She said, "No, no, no, no, no. What you need is HRT."

Those magic tablets eventually changed my life.

I'm not so sure if it worked immediately, because the problem was I was going through a divorce. So to this day I'm a little confused as to what was menopause and what was the crap I was going through. Then I think, had I not been going through the menopause, would it have been better? Would it be worse? Did I have an excuse? Did I not? I honestly can't tell you.

So, I was going through menopause, divorce, moving house and death. I say death because divorce is a death; it's the death of the life of a marriage. But you're also going through the loss of your youth. And you're mourning both of those things. I was also going through the humiliation of seeing it all in the media and my husband with someone who represented who I used to be: fun, carefree, no responsibilities. I can stand back now and dissect it and understand, but at the time I was in a complete and utter visceral fog, which I had difficulty explaining to anyone.

How did I get through it all? I think it was self-preservation. Necessity comes into it. One thing that is true of me is that I earn my living by performing, by being in the limelight. So if I wanted to carry on working, I didn't have time for this. I just couldn't have sweaty moments. I couldn't not be able to function. I couldn't hide behind a desk. The show had to go on.

I believe a hugely important element in getting through the menopause is simply to tackle your own health. Fitness and diet has to be a huge part of it. Your own health has to be put to the top of the to-do list, instead of wandering about somewhere down at the bottom. We will MOT our car before we MOT ourselves.

But also, for me, there was a little bit of vanity – and let's not underestimate that, because it's all part of our mental wellbeing. It's part of our makeup. You make the best of what you've got.

I remember once, when I was having a divorce meltdown – it was two o'clock in the afternoon and I was still looking wrecked in my pyjamas. I rang my mum and I was a snivelling wreck on the floor. I couldn't see the wood for the trees, and she said to me, "Are you dressed?" I mumbled. She said, "You have to do this. Get in the shower. Blow dry your hair." She knew that would take me at least half an hour. "Put some makeup on. Get dressed properly and call me back."

I did it and it made a difference. You have to really take hold of yourself, and you must make sure you don't let the little things drop. Keep the show on the road.

I am now on body-identical, not bioidentical, HRT. I had a bad run-in with the bioidentical HRT. I'd been trying them for a little while and struggling with them, and then, one day, I arrived at an event that I was presenting, not feeling quite right. I thought, There's really something the matter with me.

I felt terrified. I had to go into this room, get changed, and when I got there, I absolutely fell apart. I could feel my head start to sweat, my makeup was dripping off my face, it was not good. How was I going to face all these people?

Obviously, I had to pull myself together. I had no choice, but immediately afterwards I went straight to Dr Louise Newson. She had been part of a panel on the menopause run by the charity Wellbeing of Women. I had chaired the event at late notice because Andrea McLean was unable to make it. To this day I thank the universe for this chain of events. Straight away Louise told me to get off the bioidentical products, she did blood tests and prescribed me body-identical HRT that put me back on track within two weeks. I breathed a huge sigh of relief. HRT makes a difference to your skin, your hair, your demeanour, weight – just everything. It really, really does and I think I'll stay on it for the rest of my life: there's no reason to come off it as far as I'm concerned.

Louise is an amazing woman who has dedicated her professional life to educating women on the menopause. Whenever any of my friends ask me for help – I am surrounded by friends who are younger than me – I send all of them to Louise.

I don't have any symptoms now – because I'm religious, obviously, about taking my Oestradiol gel and my progesterone tablets, and testosterone cream.

Another issue with the menopause is that I have been diagnosed with osteopenia. I discovered this purely by accident about ten years ago because I was doing a television show and I had to go for a medical. They had the equipment for a DEXA test at the clinic I attended. It measures your bone density and the doctor said, "Do you want one while we're here?"

I now have a DEXA test once a year to keep a check on it. Early diagnosis can arrest the situation, as can tweaks to your diet and exercise regime; weight-bearing exercises being one tweak, along with taking a good daily dose of Vitamin D. The drop in oestrogen levels during the menopause decreases bone density by about 10 per cent. The test is something you can do through your GP, or you can go privately; if you do it's just under £200. Osteopenia is the downside of having a life of being light, as it means your bones have never had to work that hard because you're not carrying a lot of weight around, so it doesn't regenerate in the same way. HRT, again together with lifestyle choices, makes a big difference. Who wants to be the one of the one-in-two women getting fractures due to low bone density?

Now I make sure I take good quality Vitamin D, morning and night. I try to the best of my ability to make sure I go round with weights. I do Pilates. Basically I just move. I'm a great believer that if you do everyday movement correctly, you don't need to go to the gym that much. I trained in classical ballet, so there's enough muscle memory there. I bang on to my friends about the Alexander technique. We weren't put on this earth with Virgin Active; we used our body because we walked, we carried things, we used our feet and our fingers correctly.

I do believe in the word energy and the idea of good energy, moving around your body. Keep yourself energised. I'm not a stroller. I stride out. There are two things we all do every day, but not many of us do them properly, and that's walk and breathe. I've got ankle weights on now and I relish picking things up!

I am a great believer in counting my blessings. Outside of my health (touch wood), one of my blessings is my three amazing step-daughters who are in my life, every day of my life, and I have a great relationship with them. I am very much at peace with the fact that I didn't give birth to them.

We have very open conversations and I'll definitely prepare them for the menopause. I won't wait for them to ask. That's the thing, everybody's always waiting for people to ask – but you don't ask unless you're in trouble.

A while back one of my step-daughters was living with me and she said, "On your way home, can you pick me up some Tampax?" So I went into the supermarket and picked up some Tampax and a newspaper. Thinking, Oh, I haven't done this in such a long time. And as I went to the checkout, I put them down on the counter for all to see, and I felt I was saying, "Hey, I'm still ovulating, folks. Look at me. Tampax. Look, hey!" It was a funny moment.

We have, as a culture, started to talk about the menopause now. What has happened lately, in the last few years, is monumental. The sisters, those who are out there paving the way by talking about it, are doing it so that our daughters, my step-daughters who are all in their twenties, will never have to go through it unprepared.

Of course, our problems are never over. When we've got our heads around the menopause, we then have to get our heads round generally ageing, which is another little collection of problems and emotions we have to navigate. We're women, we don't want to see our hair getting thinner, we don't want to see our skin starting to have sun spots and wrinkles. If I had a pound for every woman who's said to me, "I don't want to be thirty or forty again. I want to be me, but I want the skin I had then..."

I do feel we need to change our attitudes to ageing. It's not we who judge ourselves, it's other people – but we've done the judging as well. If I said to you, "Think of a woman in her forties," you would immediately have a picture of someone in their forties. If I say, "She's in her sixties," then you have a different picture. I'm sixty. Now I'm not so sure I can deal with that picture; the picture that even I have of a person in their sixties isn't me – it's somebody else.

What you learn is that on the other side of the menopause, you do start to regenerate, and you enter what the Japanese call your Second Spring. But this one is about your mind. Youth isn't in a pot of cream. Youth is in your mind. Youth is about widening your horizons. It's about saying, I've got nothing to stop me now. No excuses.

Other cultures do embrace ageing. They embrace the wise. They don't see it as a door shutting, they see it as a door opening to a freedom that we didn't have when we were menstruating, that we didn't have because of children, life, family. We need to embrace that freedom and be a little bit selfish about it. There's nothing wrong with vanity and being a little bit selfish because you can see your mortality. You have more airmiles behind you than in front of you, so grab them – cherish, savour and enjoy every single one of them.

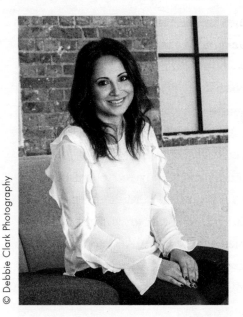

Shahzadi Harper

Menopause doctor

"Menopause is a diversity issue. I have found it very frustrating that the face of menopause is very white and middle class."

Dr Shahzadi Harper, 49, is a menopause doctor who runs her own specialist clinic in London. The daughter of a Muslim Pakistani bus driver, she is keen to change the mostly white face of menopause. It was when she found herself in a dark place, suffering from perimenopause symptoms following the loss of her father and the break-up of a difficult marriage, that she found her "calling", to listen and optimise wellbeing, both physical and psychological, for those going through this stage in life.

~

One of the things I want to do is to show women in midlife that it's not the end of life; you can have new beginnings, and you can start a new business like I did, setting up my menopause clinic. I did all that in my perimenopause, after coming out of a horrible acrimonious divorce, at a time when the chips were really down.

Menopause is a diversity issue. I have found it very frustrating that the face of menopause is very white and middle class. Firstly, I'm not white. Secondly, whereas now technically I am middle class, I haven't come from a middle-class beginning. I've wanted to show that menopause affects people, different ethnicities, slightly differently. We live in a multicultural Britain and we need to be aware of it.

I'm from a traditional Muslim Pakistani family. My dad was a bus driver. My mum was a stay-at-home mum but a very strong woman. There are no academics in my background or my extended family. No one we knew had gone to university. And so, when I got my A level results, my dad was very happy.

But he still felt he had to go to his older brother, who is also like a father figure to my dad because of the age gap, and ask him permission: "Can I send her to university?"

My uncle and I were really close. And he said, "Of course you can. But we can trust you, can't we? Just remember you're going there to study." He said that because of boys and the fact that I was going to have an arranged marriage.

I got engaged the month after I graduated and I got married six months later in an arranged marriage. I ended up living with my husband's parents and this was up in Manchester and he was quite male chauvinistic. And it was sad because I became a shadow of myself.

They didn't want me to work. But I thought, I haven't fought this hard to get to university to give it up. And then I fell pregnant. When my daughter was fifteen months old, I couldn't take it anymore. The marriage was horrible. His mother never talked to me. He undermined my self-esteem and I lost my confidence.

After my daughter was born I went back to work when she was four months old, and all I kept thinking was I need to save up a pot of money before I can leave because my parents can't give me money, because my background is not one of wealth. I just needed to create a little pot, so I could leave him.

That was what I did.

I ended up getting a job in Oxford as a GP registrar and training as a GP. I'm not going to deny it, I was little bit resentful, a little bit unhappy that my career, my life, my finances weren't falling into place. After I divorced my first husband, I was on my own for most of the time. I brought my daughter up. When she was sixteen, I thought I should really look into the next stage of my life. I was a partner in a practice at that time.

I went on a dating site that my friend encouraged me to go on and I met my future husband. It was a whirlwind. He whisked me off my feet. We got married a year later, but he was basically just a white version of the first one, controlling and narcissistic. But I was under his spell; it felt good that someone was taking care of me. The wedding was at Blenheim Palace, all bells and whistles.

And then, less than three years later, we split. I don't think he could cope with my sadness at losing my father and needing my family. He wanted me all to himself. But the good thing about it, the positive to come out of it, was I moved from Oxford to London and I'd always felt that London was a place in which I could be me.

And I could be me.

I had some dark patches in those years, and it all coincided with my own hormonal change. I was forty-four years old, and I could feel hormones were changing, but there was so little information out there.

I knew something wasn't right. The weight was increasing. I've always had issues with my weight. I can just look at croissants and it piles on top of me. It was the tiredness too. I remember being on my cross-trainer, but I was so tired, I was closing my eyes and doing it. Also, my joints ached. I felt like an old lady in the mornings!

One of my problems during the break-up of my second marriage was that even though for most of my adult life I've been on my own, single mum, bought houses, bought cars, paid my bills, managed all my finances, I'd given my power to my ex-husband, because he was a financial planner. So he had taken all that off me and managed it. There was a part of me that was like, oh finally somebody's looking after me. I became so dependent without even realising it.

When we split there were some difficult times. I can't believe how dependent I felt on him and, suddenly, it was almost like learning to walk all over again. How do I pay these bills? All of these things I had done before, he had taken charge of and put them under his company. And just as the whirlwind had begun, it ended. He literally cut me off.

Following that, I worked for a year as a maternity locum. In that time, I upped my skills, and I met Nick Panay, the menopause specialist and gynaecologist. I said to him, "I really want to do some menopause work. Can I work for you in your clinic?"

And that's what I did. But I remember one day I was walking down Harley Street to his clinic and I was a little bit unhappy because it was pouring down with rain and they'd only booked one patient in with me ... And I thought to myself, by the time I get there, go home, is it worth it? I saw a sign was up for rooms to rent and literally in less than forty-eight hours, I'd got them. I didn't really think too much about how it would work. I thought, It's now or never, what have you got to lose? You've been talking about this for years. Just go for it and believe in yourself.

I was in perimenopause. I felt like I was constantly in PMT mode. My marriage had broken down and, with that, my vision for my future, my old age. I did hit some dark patches during that divorce. I remember thinking I could walk in front of a bus. My daughter had started university, so I thought, I've done my bit for her.

The other thing was I felt I hadn't really grieved my father, because when he died we'd moved to London to set up the house and I hadn't really stopped to take a breath to think. My ex had his Christmas lunch just weeks after my father had passed away. I didn't want to put any makeup on, I didn't want to have any dinner, but I did it because I was the wife of a CEO. So I hadn't stopped. I hadn't paused to think, How do I feel? I'd gone back to work after a week and a half.

My daughter and I have a very funny, fractious relationship. We're opposites in a way, but when I split up with my ex in 2017, on my following birthday, in the card, she said, "Mum, it's your time to shine."

I thought, Yeah. These men come into my life and all they do is take my sparkle away, take my shine away. They con me.

And I just thought, This time around, whoever I meet, it's going to be on my terms. I'm not going to be that timid Muslim Pakistani girl who just is grateful to be with somebody. I thought, I'm going to do it my way. And if they're not up to what I want then it's out, you know. So I did, I did do that.

Women talk about feeling invisible at this time in life. After that break-up, I thought, I'm not ready to be invisible. I still have a lot of living and giving to do.

I'm still on my hormonal journey. It's not over. I think for me it's probably going to last for a long time. Here we are in middle age, or midlife – I don't really like the term middle age – and as women we can feel in some way stronger. Maybe we've got shorter tethers in the sense that we're not going to put up with things. We've put up with so much for so long that we sometimes say, "Well, what have we got to lose?" A confidence can come out of it.

For me, I also got to that point in my life where I thought, I want to have sex and I'm not going to feel guilty for it. I'm not going to have that Muslim guilt in my head. If I want to meet somebody, I'm just going to do it.

I now also drink champagne. (I never used to drink before.) Some peri- or menopausal women say to me, "Can I drink?" I always say, "Moderately. It's all about moderation. The alcohol can make your hot flushes worse, your anxiety worse. But it's all about moderation."

I think not enough information is out there to explain to women that it's not you, it's your hormones. Relationships end or are impacted. I've seen so many women who are thinking about career moves, or leaving their jobs. Personally, if I hadn't set up my clinic, if I'd stayed within the NHS, I don't know if I could have coped with my hormones, with those days when you can't sleep so well, when you're awake at five in the morning.

> "We've put up with so much for so long that we sometimes say, "Well, what have we got to lose?"

I'd been in the NHS for over twenty years, so I was feeling a bit of burnout. I know we've been clapping for the NHS lately [during the Covid-19 lockdown], but they're not always very kind to their own and don't understand how menopause can affect your career and that you may need some flexibility. There are maternity policies, but there are no menopause policies to help women at the other end of reproductive life. You can't say to your GP partners in a practice, "Hey look, I want to start at ten o'clock with my patients rather than half-eight because I've got to travel in from London and I don't want to feel that extra anxiety of coming in at a set time." They don't understand perimenopause.

We also really need to look at menopause through a diversity lens. In India, for someone of my ethnic origin, the average age of menopause is forty-six-and-a-half years old. But here in the UK it's fifty-one and when somebody like me at forty is having hormonal changes, employers might think, Oh, they're too young. And from a fertility point of view, women should be told earlier on so they can factor it in with planning pregnancies.

The other thing is that social class makes a huge difference to your menopause experience and how early it happens for you. The lower class you are, the earlier it comes along. I'm very much about equality and fairness, even though I've got a private clinic. We need to understand that social deprivation has a huge part to play. If you're a smoker, if you've not had any children, it tends to come along earlier.

I think for my mum the menopause was a very difficult journey because she moved to this country when she was twenty-eight and she is the big sister in her family, so she had no elder, no female relative. Her mother had died, so she didn't have her to turn to. My mum is a very bright woman – her arithmetic, her mental agility, her coping, all of that was excellent. That deteriorated. It was strange to see this woman, who was so capable, not locking the bathroom door because she was panicky and anxious; this woman who would go and stand out in the snow because she was so hot; this woman who had this sharpness of mind, such mental agility, whose mental agility fell off a cliff.

She's got dementia now. That was also another factor that got me thinking about menopause. Five years ago I was saying to people, "I know that perimenopause has a factor in dementia. We just haven't got the studies yet, but I'm sure they will come out." And now many experts are talking about HRT's positive effects on dementia and that maybe women with a family history of dementia should be considering HRT in their perimenopause.

For me, I thought the last thing I want is to lose my brain power because that's the thing that makes me who I am. And for my mother it wasn't just that her mental agility and concentration deteriorated, it was also her pelvic floor. Obviously she had eight children and that was a factor, but no one said to her it could be that your oestrogen levels are low.

From that moment she declined. Since the loss of my father it's gone down even more. It was the anxiety, the panic, the memory changes that happened, which were the big factors with my mother. They scared me as well.

I'm forty-nine now. I'm on HRT. I take oestrogen and I'm one of those progesterone-sensitive people so I cycle my progesterone. I don't like to take it monthly. I take some testosterone as well. For me I found that was the missing piece of the jigsaw. It just gives energy really. When you're on oestrogen and progesterone you're kind of content, you're ticking along. Everything is nice. And personally I don't like that word "nice". I like to think I'm a bit more spicy than that and testosterone added the spice.

I still get some anxiety at times and I've never been this anxious person. Sometimes I get overwhelmed, worried about the future and can't sleep. But then sleep and anxiety are interlinked.

The other thing I've noticed is that I'm more emotional. I cry a bit more easily. One woman said to me, "You're the best thing that has happened to me in lockdown. Because I wouldn't have bothered to contact anyone." It brought tears to my eyes, which it would not have done ten years ago.

I often think people look at me now and don't understand where I've come from. The Black Lives Matter protests really made me reflect on who I was because I'd forgotten. I now live such a privileged life compared to where I came from and I often want to share that journey with people because I want to give them hope – particularly younger girls, younger women of my ethnicity. That's why I want to mix up menopause to show different faces, different colours – because all women go through this.

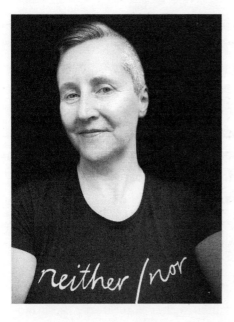

Tania Glyde

Psychotherapist

"It feels as if menopause has pulled me back through time to the age of about ten, when I was creative, imaginative, scientific, and felt pre-formed in terms of gender and sexuality."

Tania Glyde (pronouns they/she) is a psychotherapist/counsellor in private practice in London, specialising in working with Gender, Sex and Relationship Diverse clients, with a special interest in sexology. They have been researching the queer experience of menopause and how therapists and other healthcare practitioners can better support their LGBTQ+ clients and patients. Tania is the author of two novels and a memoir, and has been a journalist, broadcaster and performer.

~

I decided to research the LGBTQ+ experience of menopause after a number of conversations with queer friends. There was a sense of menopausal queers having to take a very deep breath before going to the doctor. It can be bad enough coming out as lesbian or bi – bringing gender variance into the mix potentially adds a further level of stress, with the risk of the doctor not getting it at all. On the plus side, some nonbinary people were looking forward to being prescribed testosterone by their gender clinic as it would hopefully mitigate the side effects of menopause.

One thing many LGBTQ+ folks report is just how heteronormative (and cisnormative) the public and media narrative around menopause is (via the assumption that it's only women it happens to), and how incredibly clichéd. Depressing cartoons about night sweats and cats. Worn out "battle of the sexes" humour. Mass panic over weight gain and not being able to have PIV (penis-in-vagina) sex to please your husband. The vagina must be kept available at all costs!

There is an essential ageism and misogyny around the idea that menopause is uniformly tragic, which seems to reinforce the infantilisation of older people. And the negative response to menopause also represents a major failure of mainstream sex education. If the only sex you've ever had has been PIV, with perhaps a bit of "foreplay" beforehand, menopause is likely to hit you very hard. Queer and kinky folks may experience the same bodily symptoms, but for these groups physical intimacy generally has a far wider remit from the start.

However, pink-themed gendered leaflets, for example, and constant references to male partners, can be alienating – and may keep some queer folks away from getting the help they need.

I did my research because there is almost nothing out there about the LGBTQ+ experience of menopause. Someone might have an okay experience seeking help, but they may also experience systemic ageism, misogyny (where applicable), homophobia, biphobia or transphobia. Asexuals may have to deal with all sorts of unnecessary questions and assumptions, too.

And the confusion about what is going on in our bodies can

start early, no matter how you identify. So many of us don't know when our perimenopause started because we were never told about it. With hindsight, my own menopause timeline stretches back to my late thirties. Having been clockwork-regular all my life, my periods started to become irregular when I was about thirty-nine, in 2005. Previously, I always knew exactly when they were coming, but I got a shock the day I went out dancing in a white outfit and my period came early. After a few more unpredictable incidents, I knew I couldn't rely on my body clock anymore and started keeping tampons in my bags and coats. But I had no idea there was a reason for this.

Was that the start of peri? Maybe, but I had also had some gynae issues for at least a year before that, which were misdiagnosed for ages, and I now wonder if that was actually the beginning.

I can say that the history of my menopause, like millions of others, is (at least during the early years) a history of being poorly treated by doctors. I am sad to say this, as more recently I have had good experiences.

I should say, first off, that there is an anomaly in my medical records – I had a stroke in 2008 aged forty-one, which is technically a contraindication for HRT. I got this "fact" so embedded in my brain that I didn't actually seek HRT for a while and was quite scared of it.

Aged about forty-three, I knew something was changing in me – I was low energy, kind of depressed, but differently from previously in my life. I had been reading about people taking testosterone in middle age and I tried to talk to a GP about getting a hormone test, but I was told, "We don't do hormone tests just because someone is feeling a bit down." I had no idea how to argue with that because I didn't know perimenopause was a thing.

A year later, at forty-four, I realised I was starting to struggle with my left and right (previously perfect). I started to wonder about hormonal changes and asked another GP for a test. This time I was given one, but when it came back, the GP told me that the "normal range" (that dreaded phrase that really ought to be used with far more care) was so wide that she could not tell me whether I was in menopause or not. Again, I went home none the wiser and without the baseline information to argue from.

I started to have mood swings that caused me to think I was going mad, a phrase you will often hear from people in perimenopause. Looking back, they certainly caused some challenges in my life. During this time, I had a number of gynaecological issues and consequent interactions with the healthcare system. As I remember, not a single practitioner mentioned menopause. Although I was memorably asked by one young doctor if I was "still having sex"!

At forty-eight, I started to have hot flushes. They first happened when I was with a client – my glasses were steaming up and at first I thought it was erotic countertransference! I put two and two together and went back to another doctor, who did a test. When the test came back, she told me the results were "within the normal range" and dismissed me. I asked her what on earth these disturbing heat spikes could be. Was I fighting a virus? "Well, I don't know!" she said, very rudely, and sent me on my way. Yet again, I didn't have the knowledge to argue with this.

I was left with an increasing sense of being gaslighted by the medical profession.

The following year I went back because the hot flushes were getting worse. We are now in 2015, the year the NICE guidelines for GPs about menopause came out. I got a very nice doctor, who said I could not have HRT because of my stroke (while not looking more closely at my notes), and said that at forty-nine and a half I was a "bit young" for menopause! Apparently fifty is the literal magic age that everything needs to be judged against. She also said that, as I had been having flushes for six months, I "should be done with them by the end of the year". Here I am, five years of hot flushes later!

So I went away and dealt with it. My periods stopped mid-2015.

It felt very hard to get clarity. In 2016 I started to get terrible anxiety which sometimes kept me awake all night. It sometimes manifested as being halfway to falling asleep, but then being jerked awake by a sharp sense of dread and fear.

My sleep had not been good for a while, and it got worse. I did not connect all this with menopause because I did not realise they were connected. The anxiety continued, and so did the flushes, as well as other symptoms, and by 2017, aged fifty-one, I was feeling desperate. All this was happening to me on top of doing a very intense and hands-on sex-educator training.

As you can imagine, the combined effect of these confusing and debilitating symptoms was not great. It affected my relationships and my life in general. I returned to see yet another doctor, an excellent GP, who had a good look at my records.

For a start, the previous doctor had not told me the truth – my results had clearly showed I was in menopause. Better news was that the stroke I'd had in 2008 was an arterial dissection, not a blood clot. It's the latter kind which is contraindicated for HRT. After discussion, my GP decided this was safe enough and started me on HRT in pill form.

It took a while to get the dose right. I tried Femoston Conti at a lower dose and then a higher one. A full dose got rid of all the physical symptoms, which was great, but unfortunately it made me depressed, like clockwork, about thirty minutes after taking them. I then tried Tibolone (a synthetic steroid that the body can convert into hormones), but it didn't have much effect, and showed none of its fabled androgenic properties – i.e. improved libido. So I moved onto patches, Evorel Conti. A whole patch made me depressed again, so I cut them into two-thirds. It was not perfect but okay enough and better than nothing. Next, after doing some research, I started asking for testosterone, and my GP referred me to a specialist clinic.

Then, aged fifty-two, after ten months on HRT, I was diagnosed with breast cancer. It was caught early, and I had surgery and radiotherapy, but it meant I had to come off the HRT immediately. And my specialist NHS menopause clinic appointment took so long to come round that by the time I got there I had the cancer diagnosis, and they said they could not give me the testosterone, as the body converts it to oestrogen.

How did I feel about all these symptoms? What I felt was varying levels of compartmentalised distress and irritation. Until the later stages, there was little sense of "this is menopause", so I felt very much dissociated from the idea that it was menopause that was doing this. My feelings about menopause are also framed by my experiences of being gaslighted by the healthcare system.

What I also experienced was a sense of my own inadequacy, that I couldn't somehow do it "better". I think the narrative of skinny celebrity women in the media having massages and herbal blah blahs in Thailand after getting specially tailored hormones from private doctors could probably do with an upgrade. I don't knock going private – many save up and go out of desperation when the NHS won't help – but most people have to work throughout their lives and may not be able to retire ever. Many

> The narrative of skinny celebrity women in the media having massages and herbal blah blahs in Thailand after getting specially tailored hormones from private doctors could probably do with an upgrade.

menopausal people I have spoken to would give up work tomorrow if they could, and are exhausted from running on empty. But giving up work is not an option for most.

In fairness to the system, for me breast cancer and menopause got wrapped around each other – recovering from the treatment for one exacerbated the other. It felt simply unfair that I had to stop taking medication that was at least partially helping. I started my MA just after finishing radiotherapy, which I have no regrets about and am very pleased I did, but it was a lot one after the other.

At fifty-four, five years in, I am getting my energy back. Menopause is like a slow dark explosion happening in the middle of your life. While I feel as if I have lost something, I can also see a new and exciting way forward.

Personally, I have been lucky with medical practitioners regarding my bisexuality in this context. I still notice a tendency towards assuming heterosexuality and calling everyone "ladies" – I really wish healthcare people would stop this and I have been calling it out more.

My menopause study was originally intended to focus on the experiences of the queer menopausal client in therapy, but I wanted to find out about my participants' experiences in a wider system, so my questions included a long section on general healthcare.

I found there was an overall sense of a lack of knowledge about menopause, and "you don't know what you don't know". Several reported their own mothers being very ill with it and having to take long periods off work, but it was something hidden under the table. The impression they had was that menopause is when you become "an old lady".

There was an overwhelming sense of therapists and other health-care practitioners making assumptions from a top-down position, i.e. acting as if they knew the queer menopausal person better than the person knew themselves. In fact, it is the queer menopausal patient who ends up having to educate the practitioner. One genderqueer participant had the particularly distressing experience of being interrogated about their genitals.

The non-consensual writing of prescriptions was a feature of some accounts – with the doctor either pushing antidepressants on someone, or HRT, without a proper discussion.

These challenging experiences came on top of negative past experiences of microaggressions, prejudice and exclusion, which were in turn further compounded by having to negotiate confusing and distressing symptoms, such as insomnia and anxiety. Lack of information about menopause meant that some people thought they were going mad, and these symptoms in perimenopause could interact badly with existing diagnoses, such as ADHD or bipolar.

Participants who were considering transition at the same time as menopause had the difficult task of performing for two sets of gatekeepers, GPs and gender clinics. At the GPs taking care not to mention gender (or risk being sent away), and at the gender clinic taking care not to mention menopause (or risk being told they are not trans enough and being sent away).

It's also very possible that some transmasculine people are not getting help because even the word menopause triggers dysphoria in them. One of my participants found their gender clinic to be very helpful around this, by taking care not to use the word, but this meant that they didn't realise what the symptoms of oestrogen deficiency are.

There were also positives. Many were glad to see the end of periods and fertility, though some, even though they had never wanted children, needed to take some time to reflect on the loss of this capacity. There was a general sense that there are many benefits to being queer – you are, to some extent, protected against the patriarchal demands made of cis-het women, and the obligation to perform certain roles (and narrow forms of penis-focused sex) in order to be seen as acceptable.

I'm aware I've said a lot of negative things about my menopause experience. I've said them because they needed saying and because I felt so unheld. The medical system can be stressful and leave a bad memory, and sometimes trauma. Plus, systemic ageism means that anything connected with the ageing process may cause us to deny or try to repress it. Actually, though, this menopause journey has many upsides to it. No more periods and no more fertility, for a start!

One of the most striking things about my own experience is that it feels as if menopause has pulled me back through time to the age of about ten, when I was creative, imaginative, scientific, and felt pre-formed in terms of gender and sexuality. I was one of those only children who always felt like an alien. I loved cars and building things as much as I loved dolls, and I just kind of did my own thing.

This sense of "returning to original me" has been powerful. In life, like so many people, I have often felt as if I was going along with things just to stay safe. This feeling has been changing for me, for quite a while now. If you asked me my gender identity today I might say genderqueer. I have been moving towards using a "they" pronoun for a few years now, not necessarily linked to menopause. I am not repulsed by the identity "woman", and nor do I wish to distance myself from that part of my life, but now it feels as if I am on a fast-moving train, waving goodbye to the woman still standing on the platform.

At around forty I began to become invisible to men in the street. If I lost some weight, I might take on a hazy outline and be noticed. Two years ago I began to cut my hair shorter. I got some new glasses and started to become less invisible. During the Covid-19 lockdown, I stopped colouring my hair and now have a silver/grey buzzcut. There is something I am loving about being less subject to the aggression from men (and women) that I experienced when younger. But mainstream society also desexes you at this age.

In the queer and kinky community, there can be more leeway around age, and age-gap relationships, and you may be written off less than in cis-het vanilla culture.

It's important to use inclusive language as a reminder that not everyone with ovaries is a woman, and may be trans or nonbinary. We need more research into intersex experiences of menopause. And, going wider, the experiences of people of colour, because so far the "gold standard" for menopause research has been white American women.

It's also important to remember that menopause is biopsychosocial. Put simply, it's concerned with the mind, the body and the society around you. The social aspects mean that the narrative is not confined to people with ovaries. All bodies can undergo some sort of hormonal transition in midlife. This means that trans women can also experience feelings akin to menopause, whether due to the ageing process, having to come off hormones (because of, for example, the current HRT shortage in 2020, which is affecting so many people), or the effects of certain medications. One of my research participants was a trans woman; more studies on menopausal-type experiences in this group would be very welcome.

Ultimately, I don't think the menopause is bad or good; it's a life phase. However, the way it's dealt with, through a lens of ageism, ableism and prejudice, means that many people suffer unnecessarily. The end of fertility for many will be celebrated, especially if they come from somewhere where providing children is demanded as part of a social contract. Many have terrible periods, and so celebrate the end of them.

I think the idea that it's a terrible tragedy may have Western roots and treating it that way colludes with the idea that women and all people with ovaries should feel terrible about themselves. The obsession with youth I think is global, but in the West the idea of ageing as tragic and repulsive is particularly embedded in how we are encouraged to see ourselves.

One thing we all need to learn, queers included, is that hormones are not gendered! We have these terrible binary ideas that testosterone is the man hormone, all chest beating and macho, and oestrogen is the woman hormone, all squeaky voice and softness. This is rubbish. All bodies need testosterone, oestrogen and progesterone to function. Different levels, sure, but they are all there. We have all been tripped up by this nonsense and it is preventing some people getting help. A woman will not be masculinised by a low dose of T, and a man will not be feminised by a bit of oestrogen. It's possible for older transmasculine people on testosterone to have oestrogen deficiency, which means some people may be suffering but not getting help.

We need more genetic studies of hormones to really understand how they work in different people. More people need to be able to access hormones and we need to truly understand the health factors in taking them versus the health factors in not taking them. The bottom line is that reduced oestrogen production in the body is a potential health issue and you cannot get away from that. I often wonder if we should call menopause "Oestrogen Deficiency Syndrome" and then perhaps it would be taken more seriously.

PAIN

(noun)

A highly unpleasant physical or
emotional sensation. It hurts.

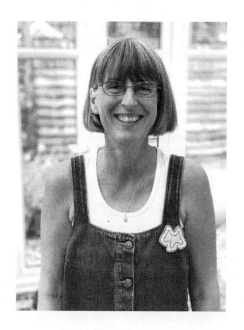

Jane Lewis

Vaginal atrophy
campaigner

*"The burning was like sitting
on a bonfire and if you bent
over you felt like you were
going to split open."*

Jane Lewis's preoccupation was horses until one day she found the torment of vaginal atrophy made it impossible to sit on one. She was a florist until menopausal befuddlement and the distraction of pain made her worry she might miss a wedding. Then she started to research her condition, wrote and self-published *Me & My Menopausal Vagina*, discovering to her horror that too many women are living in this agony.

~

Vaginal atrophy is the taboo of taboos. Menopause is taboo, but vaginal problems are taboo taboo.

I was about fortyish when sex became very slightly painful. I now admin an online group of a few thousand women and what I find there is that the very first symptoms are either that smear tests start hurting or sex gets slightly painful. But it's so slight that you ignore it.

Then for me it was in my mid-forties when the symptoms started to accelerate. I got really itchy on my legs, on the shins, and all my mucosal membranes. I got this condition called runny eye, which is actually dry eyes. I had a dry burning mouth, itchy ears, sore nose, and then the vulva problems.

It's called vaginal dryness, but for me especially it was more external, around the vulva area. There are actually thirteen symptoms that can come from vaginal dryness and I had most of them.

I'm fifty-four in August, but I'm still considered perimenopausal because I still have follicles in my ovaries and we can't entirely regulate my hormones with HRT. It is a very big myth that vaginal dryness only affects postmenopausal women. Among my online group, I would say we are around half perimenopausal still having regular periods and half postmenopausal. So it is happening in perimenopause.

A lot of women don't realise they've got the problem because they don't associate bladder problems as part of it. Bladder issues and repeat UTIs, getting up in the night all the time, leakage, are part of it as well. And vaginal atrophy can put women off going for smears. One GP did a local audit for women over forty-eight, asking, "Why haven't you turned up?" And they all said because it's too painful. They were given local oestrogen for about six weeks and they all came and had a pain-free smear.

I knew from fairly early on what my condition was. The problem was convincing those around me because I was still so young. Only now are medics starting to acknowledge they're seeing women who are having it younger. In fact, women were always having it younger than many people think, it's just that often it was misdiagnosed as thrush – and thrush is one of the most over-diagnosed women's issues out there.

The other thing was I became very down, very low. But if your vulva is very sore – imagine having a bees' nest or burning between your legs 24/7, or your old episiotomy scar starts to split, its surface tearing really easily – that is enough to make you have depression.

I was so low I got suicidal – the pain was so bad. The burning was like sitting on a bonfire and if you bent over you felt like you were going to split open. I just got to a point where I couldn't see the woods for the trees.

Also, I was a horse rider and had a horse of my own. The world of horses is a very social as well as physical thing. I was extremely physically fit. Sadly, my horse was put down around the same time as I was getting the extreme symptoms and that social life stopped overnight. Now, even if I wanted to have another horse, I couldn't go back. It's just not possible for me to sit on one. And I've completely lost my nerve around horses.

It was a big lifestyle that literally shut down overnight. With it went the smell of the horse, and the fact I'd be outside six or seven hours a day. A lot of ladies suffer in different ways. For some their life is cycling and cyclists can really suffer. Suddenly they can't bear their bike saddles. Some do find a better saddle, some don't. A lot of the ladies in my group can't wear their gym clothes anymore because they're too tight and get too sweaty.

My work was affected, too. I had my own business as a wedding florist and it was really busy. Some years I had up to sixty weddings a year and I nearly forgot two because I was so distracted in my mind with the pain. I couldn't juggle anymore. I had to call it a day because I knew that one day I was actually going to forget the bride's wedding. I've got befuddlement as a menopause symptom on its own. I really struggle.

I'm now on HRT, and it is working but, because I am still what's called perimenopausal, and still have periods, my own hormones are still going up and down. I'm not pushing HRT in my book, but I need HRT without a doubt, just for my vagina and bladder areas. Without it, I probably wouldn't be here.

I didn't know anything about vaginal atrophy before I had my symptoms – yet it is something that affects most women. If you look up vaginal atrophy you'll get sites that will tell you that it affects roughly 50 per cent of postmenopausal women. Dr Louise Newson, whenever she does a podcast or talks about it, will say 70 per cent. And then you have a book that's called *Oestrogen Matters*, by Dr Avrum Bluming, who will say it's as much as nearly all: he believes every postmenopausal woman is experiencing it to some degree.

The average woman tends to think the menopause is just heavy periods, possibly going a little bit mad and getting hot and sweaty. We need to change that. When I was researching my condition I noticed that most of the books about the menopause touch on vaginal dryness in only an insignificant way. Yet it is one of the top symptoms out there. So I decided to write my own book, *Me & My Menopausal Vagina*. I couldn't write it myself – I just don't have the grammatical skills – but I wrote something down and I gave it to my daughter who said, "Mother, you can't put that." But it had humour and I knew I wanted humour in it, because being a sufferer I can see the humour in such a horrid condition. It became a family project and we ended up self-publishing it.

I know my vaginal problems are here for life. They can't cure it. Most of the symptoms, like hot flushes, will hopefully reduce over time, but specialists know that the vaginal problems will not. If they're not treated, they only get worse and treatment is for life. If you stop it, it comes back, and often it comes back worse and it's harder to get back on top of it.

I have to be on at least local oestrogen for life. But I have chosen to be on HRT for life simply because I have sat in a lot of talks and lectures now by medics, and I know for me personally the benefits

– to your heart, bones, everything else – far outweigh the risks. But I also know about elderly care and how, as we age, UTIs are a huge problem, including urinary sepsis, and women are prone to them through lack of oestrogen as we age. That's why I want to stay on it to keep my brain, and my pelvic-urogenital areas, healthy for as long as possible.

My husband has been amazing all along, and he never wanted me to have sex that was painful. We have it still sometimes, but it's not as it was, and I have to be careful, but he has never given me any stress at all. I've been very lucky. But there are marriages or partnerships out there that are falling apart.

We need to talk about having non-penetrative sex in menopause. We are too hung up on penetrative sex, and also for lots of us our whole vulval area and clitoris and everything is really painful and sore. Everything has to be so much more careful. You have to relax because the more painful it is, the more you tense up. I can have what I call flare-ups and the last fortnight has been really miserable. But I'm good again now and that's probably to do with my own background hormones doing things as well. It's so unpredictable.

What happens with a lot of ladies is they actually stop having sex, because sex is painful. Their pain is completely gone and so they don't think they have a problem because they don't have external pain.

Two years on from me publishing my book, things have definitely moved on. Lots of medics have read it and have admitted they didn't realise this was happening. They've changed their ways and how they talk to women about it in consultations. I've had huge support from the medical profession. I now get an awful lot of people who are talking on my public Instagram page about their problems, which eighteen months ago they wouldn't have considered doing.

The thing is that most of us women, without treatment, will go through some form of it. I did an Instagram Live two weeks ago with menopause specialist Dr Sarah Ball and we talked about local oestrogen and vaginal dryness. I said, "The number of menopausal women affected is roughly 70 per cent, isn't it?"

She said she thought that in fact there was no woman, within the ageing population, who wasn't likely to get it in some form.

> "Incontinence is treated like it's a rite of passage, something to get all giggly about when you go on a trampoline. It might be common, but it's not normal.

You only have to go into a care home to become aware of this. The main reason a woman goes into the care home is dementia or double incontinence and they are riddled with UTIs, and very unhealthy bladder, vulva and vagina. Women are sitting in pads 24/7. One of my final thoughts in the book was around elderly care, and how no one was talking about it. I've had medics who have privately messaged me since saying it's a mega problem.

We have to age. We are ageing. But if you are in pads 24/7 in a care home where there is only basic intimate care, what's going to happen? We're in for a big shock if we end up there. That's why I want to keep my brain as fit as possible, as well as my vulva-vagina area.

I want to try and be a voice for elder care. That's where I'm heading with it. I started off with vaginal dryness at my age – that's where I was. But I've opened Pandora's box. You are postmenopause for life. I want this to be made an issue.

One woman told me that her mother had had a stroke and all she could do was move her left hand. Every time she went to visit in hospital her mother's hand would go, she thought, to her stomach.

After a while, she realised it wasn't her stomach but her vulva. When she had a look she found it was raw. You've got women who are disabled going through menopause with all these issues of intimate care. With a man we can just, well, you can see if his penis or testicles are sore, can't you? But with women you need to intimately investigate and it would be inappropriate. Because where you're sore is in the nooks and crannies.

When I look back, both my grandmothers smelled of urine and you thought of it as just normal. And to wear pads is considered normal. Incontinence is treated like it's a rite of passage, something to get all giggly about when you go on a trampoline. It might be common, but it's not normal. The vast majority of women can be sorted out with a women's health physiotherapist or HRT to help the pelvic floor, or both. If you start wearing and accepting pads at fifty, it's going to cost you a lot of money and you will get repeat UTIs, and you will get soreness. You'll get nappy rash.

Dr Sarah Ball posted up the other day, saying this is a common conversation to have with a woman.

"Do you have any vagina dryness problems?"

"No."

"Do you have any bladder problems?"

"No."

"So, you're telling me you have nothing?"

"Yes."

Then she'll say, "Did you get up to the toilet last night. Do you have cystitis feelings? Do you leak?"

The patient will say, "Oh yes I have that. That's common, isn't it?"

Women dismiss it with that phrase "it's common", but it doesn't need to be common.

Once you get into the world of vaginas, you learn a lot about other conditions. I know quite a lot about other skin conditions that we can get muddled up with vaginal dryness – for instance, something called lichen sclerosus. It's important to know the difference because if lichen sclerosus isn't treated correctly, three to five per cent of cases turn to vulval cancer. It's why I make a big point of telling women that they should examine themselves, monthly, to find your normal.

Get the mirror out. A lot of women don't even know they have a vulva. They say, "My vagina itches." But unless you put your entire hand up there, it is your vulva that will be itching. A lot of women have no idea where their urethra is; some think they wee right out of the vagina, or even the clitoris. It's also really important that women don't self-treat, which we know is a big problem because of all the products that are for sale for burning, itching and soreness. Women shouldn't be putting on these products until they've looked or had it checked out because that burning, itching or soreness could actually be some other vulval condition.

I made a huge point of not being sponsored at all. I won't promote any product. Yes, I may use a product and if I mention it, it's because I have decided it works, not because someone has asked me. Because vaginal products are big money – and a lot of them have ingredients that aren't good. They are a big money-maker, and you have to be really careful when you're talking about things to do with the vagina. I see a lot of information out there that's incorrect, and I do now politely message them privately and say, what you're saying is incorrect.

When I wrote my book, I didn't tell anyone. I didn't tell my neighbour. I didn't want anyone to feel that they had to buy my book. I knew it would make some people possibly feel uncomfortable. I don't want to force it on people at all. But the book had been out two weeks and my neighbour texted me saying, "Have you written a book?" Within two weeks she had seen it recommended on Mumsnet.

I've done and said things that the old me would never have imagined. I never used to talk about vaginas in this way. My life, as I said, was horses. But I got so low I started talking about it. I found Diane Danzebrink, founder of the Menopause Support campaign, #MakeMenopauseMatter, and we were on Channel 5 together. I have no idea how I managed to get on the TV, but there I was, talking about my vagina on Channel 5!

I often think this is utterly bizarre. But I am doing it. On my Instagram I've got a few thousand followers. Some of them call me a national treasure because I have spoken about what is never being spoken about. People see me as the woman next door.

I try to come across as normal! I know I'm considered a bit eccentric and a bit potty sometimes – but we absolutely need to talk about this.

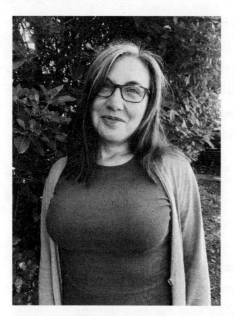

Alison
Martin-Campbell

Executive assistant

*"One of the main symptoms is
severe pain during sex.
I mean unbelievable pain,
which was one of the things
that suggested to me I had
vaginal atrophy."*

Alison Martin-Campbell, 54, is an executive assistant at the professional services firm, EY (Ernst & Young). After experiencing hot flushes,
insomnia and cystitis – the last of these so bad she ended up in hospital
– she started to share her research and tips for how to cope with the
menopause and set up the EY 40+ Network to support employees
going through midlife issues, including the menopause.

~

When I was forty-seven, I was getting recurrent bouts of cystitis, as
well as insomnia and occasional hot flushes, and I was in and out of
the doctor's repeatedly. On one occasion my symptoms were so bad
I was briefly hospitalised because the infection had taken over my
whole body. I had to take five weeks off from my work at EY. When I
was admitted to hospital, I was given a thorough examination under

anaesthetic to check if there was anything seriously wrong with me. But I was told they could find nothing wrong.

I remember, while I was in hospital, I spoke to the registrar, who was a man, a highly qualified medical healthcare professional, and I said, "Do you think I'm possibly perimenopausal?"

"No," he said, "at forty-seven you're far too young."

On reflection now, of course I was perimenopausal!

I had also been suffering chronic insomnia in the years running up to this, just the most awful insomnia, which I get a lot anyway, but which was all to do with the flushes. I was having up to twenty hot flushes a night and it didn't matter what I did. I would swim regularly. I don't drink a lot of tea and coffee. I drink a lot of water. I was trying to avoid the foods you should avoid. I was at the end of my tether. And I'd also been getting all these other symptoms. I was really uncomfortable a lot of the time with a constant desire to pass water.

When that registrar told me I wasn't perimenopausal, I thought, you're wrong. So I went on the website Menopause Matters and that's where I read my symptoms and, *tick*, it seemed I had vaginal atrophy. Every woman on there who had it was describing something very similar to what I was experiencing, so I went to my own GP and said, "I think I've got vaginal atrophy." After examining me, she confirmed that I had.

Finally, I was diagnosed with a very common condition, which doesn't get talked about very much. Vaginal atrophy affects at least 50 per cent of women in the menopause. All those times I was given antibiotics for cystitis, it was actually vaginal atrophy.

Vaginal atrophy is a thinning of the vaginal walls which is obvious to a healthcare professional. You get cystitis symptoms, feel generally uncomfortable, and have a feeling like you need to wee all the time. When I started talking about it to other women, I discovered that it is really common. Those adverts on the telly for Tena Lady products? Well, this is why a lot of women have to use them.

Thinking back, the first time that sudden need to wee happened really badly to me, I was at a Halloween party, dancing to a lively song with all my friends, when all of a sudden I thought I had completely lost control of my bladder. I was thinking, Oh my God, what's happening?

This was affecting my whole life. For example, I needed to know where the toilets were wherever I was and particularly if I had to travel. Another one of the main symptoms is severe pain during sex. I mean unbelievable pain, which was one of the things that suggested to me I had vaginal atrophy. This is very, very common; nearly all my female friends who are menopausal have it. HRT and lube sorted the painful sex out! It helps with the weeing, too, but I have to say I can't drink tea at all. I think it's something to do with the tannins irritating my sphincter muscles.

I did a lot of research. I bought lots of books. I found out about things like red clover, black cohosh, HRT, all sorts of things. I started developing a crib sheet for my own reference. When I casually mentioned it to a few girlfriends, they asked me to send it to them. So I started sending it out to anyone who asked.

I was distributing my crib sheet to fellow perimenopausal and menopausal women and, as you probably know, in large corporate organisations like EY they have many supportive networks. And several of my friends said I ought to set up an EY menopause network.

My friends said, "There are so many of us suffering." And I said I would try.

So I approached Diversity and Inclusion, and they said, "Hmmm, we can't have an EY menopause network because it's too gender-specific but you can set up something that encompasses it."

So I came back with the idea of the EY 40+ network to support staff around three areas relating to middle age – health, finances and care – but as time has passed and the network has developed, the finances aspect has been dropped (particularly since the setting up of youplusmoney@uk.ey.com), and the focus of the network is now health (not just menopause) and ageing in the workplace. I do still touch on care, but as there is now also an EY Carers' Network, there is less focus on this; although I am very much aware that caring for a loved one and one's own health can be heavily connected during middle age.

With regards to health, as we get older, we get arthritis, MS, go deaf, have to care for elderly relatives. As well as my elderly parents, when I set up the network I also supported a friend who has learning difficulties, so I need to be there for him quite a lot too. As time went on, my main focus has been around ageing and care in the workplace, but the big focus of the last two years has definitely been about health and the menopause.

I had really resisted going on HRT because I'd had a really bad experience on the pill when I was young. It made me very depressed and I have a tendency to depression anyway. I was also worried about putting hormones in my body.

Finally I did go on it about two and a half years ago and I have to say it's been fantastic. I'm a vegan so I chose bioidentical hormones, made from plant proteins. I tried lots of supplements but the thing that has helped the most has definitely been the HRT. It's great for mood. Obviously with fewer flushes, I'm sleeping a lot better. The medical profession believes you can stay on it safely for at least five years and, for many women, the benefits protecting against heart disease in particular definitely outweigh the risks of certain female-specific cancers.

When I started taking HRT, it took about two or three weeks

to start to notice the difference. And I was on it for about eighteen months, and then it seemed to stop working. But this was at a time of extreme stress with my parents. I was off work. And I came off it for about three months, thinking it wasn't working. But when I came off it, I found I was so much worse. So I went back on it. And again, within about two or three weeks, it started working. And so I've been back on it now, and I just know it's the right thing for me.

There are all sorts of long-term health benefits from HRT and I think the risks around the cancers are very small. So I'll stay on it for another two years at least and then I'll review it. My mum's sister went on HRT in 1980 when she was fifty and she took it until the day she died when she was eighty-four. She said it transformed her life and she couldn't have worked without it.

I still get a couple of hot flushes a night, but two or three a night is a damn sight better than twenty a night. Lately I have been sleeping quite well. I have been doing a lot of gardening, which is wearing me out, and I've got a neighbour who's not well and, due to lockdown, is unable to walk his dog, so I have been doing this too. I feel being outside – whatever the weather – definitely helps with symptoms and mood.

The hot flushes don't have the intensity they used to have before I started taking HRT; the heat would literally start at my chest and go all the way up my neck and head. I would feel like my hair must be wringing and I must look like a greasy frying pan of fat. The more you think about what you must look like to other people, the worse it gets, because it's just stressing you.

My sleep hasn't been great over the last year, but then I was caring for my elderly parents and they both died at the beginning of this year, within three weeks of each other. That time caring for my mum and dad was very difficult. My husband and I actually moved from London to be nearer my parents two and a half years ago, because things were getting really bad. My mum had seven strokes over the course of four years and a heart attack, and my dad was not equipped to be a carer. He had behavioural issues as well as health issues. Because he was a man of a generation where the woman ran the home, he resented having to take on the role of carer and home-maker. I took over some of the domestic tasks, with visits three or four times a week.

There was also a lot of emotional stuff going on. My mum deteriorated before my eyes with each stroke and she had vascular dementia for the last few months as well, and my dad was very angry a lot of the time. So it was difficult.

I worked part-time for a number of years because of my parents' ill health. And I also had to have time off unexpectedly when I wasn't sleeping, because I was so stressed. I had to take over a lot of the running of my parents' finances. My dad didn't do computers, didn't do online banking, kept forgetting his PIN for his card for the cash machine. I took out lasting power of attorney about four years before they died. And that was actually really helpful.

One of the most difficult things was my dad getting angry. He would have a go at me and this is quite common with older people when they're upset. If they can't express their emotions, it comes out as anger. We had screaming matches.

I did get very angry myself at times. It happens – particularly when you haven't slept and you are hot-flushing and you have cystitis and you just think there isn't any part of your body that wants to behave itself. I had a lot of challenges with my dad, I have to say. But I probably wouldn't have had those screaming matches with him if I hadn't been menopausal.

I know that the stress can make the flushes come on and the insomnia. When I was in the grips of one of my worst bouts of insomnia, I actually did a crib sheet for that, which I shared with people. A lot of the issues I addressed were the obvious things: sleep hygiene, no caffeine, not too much alcohol, plenty of exercise, fresh air, all those sorts of things which sound obvious but definitely help and can have a huge positive influence on the quality of one's life.

Something that helped was upping the exercise. I know it's boring. But that's one of my bits of advice. Also, one can have a tendency to think, This is so awful, I don't want to see my friends. But actually, it's better to see your friends and keep up your relationships. I found, when I was angry or upset and thinking *nobody's going to want to talk to me*, that when I started reaching out to friends – male friends as well as female – they would say, "Just talk." And you know, it may be a cliché, but I always felt better after.

When I was at my lowest with the perimenopause symptoms about five years ago and was talking to an older very sympathetic friend she commented, "And do you honestly feel like you are going mad sometimes with all the symptoms?" And I replied that I did. She said that was completely normal but not talked about. I often quote that to friends who are struggling particularly and reassure them that the "madness" will lift.

There really is a thing called "meno-brain". I honestly forget conversations I have had and at one point thought I had dementia. But the fog has lifted and I found making lists, doing crosswords and puzzles and reading (clichéd but true!) all do help.

I didn't have kids. I married quite late in life and it wasn't an issue for me because I hadn't wanted them. So no, I didn't have that kind of, "Oh my God, I'm never gonna do that." And most of my friends don't have children either.

The menopause hasn't really changed my character. I've always been a fairly open and honest person and it didn't really occur to me not to talk about the menopause. I really am the alien in my family, because I'll talk about anything. And I'm quite an expressive person. I would just talk about it with anyone who raises it with me.

If anything, going through the menopause has given me more confidence to talk about it and raise issues. A couple of weeks ago, EY had a forum about how we were going to organise going back into the office [after the Covid-19 lockdown]. I was invited. At the end, they said, "If you've got any extra questions or points you wish to raise, stay on the line." So I did. I stayed on with the two ladies leading it.

I said, "I just want to point out, I do have a concern that we don't have enough toilets. And it's not just about going to the toilet. But when you're going through the menopause sometimes you just want to run your wrists under the cold tap. Sometimes you need to splash your face with water. Sometimes you just need to go to a booth." After I said this, they said, "Oh, yeah, we haven't thought about all of that."

> It's really important that we create menopause-friendly workplaces.

It would never have occurred to me not to say that. As I was telling them, I realised there were two men waiting to speak afterwards. But I thought, well, they've either got a girlfriend, a wife, a sister, a mother and it's good that they know it.

It's really important that we create menopause-friendly work-places. There are literally millions of women who are going to be working for that third of their life when they're either going through the actual worst bits of the menopause, right until they hopefully come out the other side of it, and they need help with that.

One big change, one good thing, is that you can joke about the menopause now. You can have a laugh about it far more now. In a light-hearted way, you can just say, "Oh, I'm having a hot flush." If

I'm in a meeting we'll laugh about it with my team, you know; it's just one of those things.

I don't think I could have done that five years ago. It's baby steps, in all honesty. If you think about periods, forty years ago, when I was a teenager, you did not discuss them at all. And now people seem to talk about them quite freely. It's not uncommon for male friends to say, "Oh, my partner won't be coming. She's got really bad period pain." Hopefully the menopause will go that way as well.

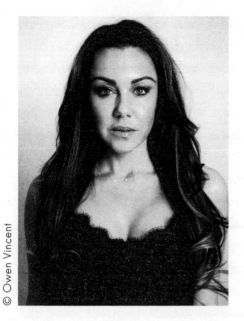

Michelle Heaton

Singer

"I was angry with the world — for a while — and then I realised everyone has their scars, whether it's physical or mental, on the inside or outside."

Michelle Heaton, 41, is a singer and a member of the pop group, Liberty X. In 2012, she had a double mastectomy after testing positive for the BRCA2 mutation gene. A family history and 35 per cent chance of getting ovarian cancer at a young age meant she made the decision to have a total hysterectomy. She is married to Hugh Hanley, CIO of My PT Hub, and has two children, Faith and AJ, and Bella their family dog. Her openness about early menopause and preventative surgery has been taboo-busting. Her book, *Hot Flush: Motherhood, the Menopause and Me*, is a ground-breaking memoir of early menopause.

~

This whole journey began when my dad found out he had the BRCA2 cancer gene. His mum and his grandma had breast and ovarian cancer in their thirties and it came to light that it had been a genetic thing. I got an automatic letter, when I was pregnant with my daughter, Faith, from the genetics department in Newcastle, the Centre of Life, saying that your dad is positive – would you like to come for a test?

I hadn't heard of it before. This is before people were talking so much about the gene, even pre-Angelina Jolie, when she opened up about her double mastectomy. I didn't know my chances. All I knew really was what my dad had told me and he knew very little. You see, for a man the risks are lower than for a woman, even though if you have the gene it is what it is – you either have it or you don't.

I put the letter in a drawer and forgot about it. Then I had my daughter, Faith, and on the day she was born, I decided to donate the cord blood. All these medical questions seemed quite confusing and fussy if I'm honest, but one stood out, and it related to hereditary genes. I wasn't sure if I could tick "have" or "don't have". I told the midwife why and in a very abrupt but compassionate way she said, "Please get the test because that little girl you're holding could have it too."

I was in bits. It never dawned on me that Faith could have it too, and I'd never know unless I got the test. It took having Faith to realise I'd be selfish if I didn't. The midwife told me a bit about BRCA2 and the genetic implications. But, in a haze while looking at Faith, I honestly can't remember a word. Within days I replied to the letter that was in the top drawer. I think it was a couple of weeks later I went to Great Ormond Street Hospital, which was a bit unnerving, because as I walked through with my healthy little girl, I realised how fortunate we were and how we could help decide our fate with this test.

It was the first step – just a blood test, but of course I cried looking down at Faith. You start to realise how serious this is when they hand you leaflets and tell you they've got counselling available if you need it.

It was about six weeks later I received a letter saying, we have your results and we recommend you bring somebody with you. I was starting to panic, but Hugh said, "It's fine, Shel, that's a normal letter but of course I will come with you anyway." So the three of us entered the same room. Our bums didn't even touch the seats before she said those words. "I'm so sorry to say you are positive."

I was holding my breath and tears in, holding Faith far too tight and she started to cry. I still get goose bumps about it now.

I don't think anything she was explaining for the next hour sunk in. She was giving advice, help, suggestions, but I didn't really hear anything. Hugh's answer to uncomfortable situations is either the gym or food. Mine's wine! So we went to Nando's, as you do. Over his meal and my glass of wine I literally carved out the next two years of my life. As a couple we decided, given the 85 per cent risk of breast cancer, I would go for a double mastectomy, reconstruction as soon as we could. Because I also had a 35 to 40 per cent risk of ovarian cancer, we decided to go for total hysterectomy, including ovary removal, too.

I had a number of reasons why I chose this path. Obviously, number one, to eliminate the risk of cancer, something that was highly likely to happen, given the information presented to me, including taking into consideration the age at which my grandma and great-grandma were diagnosed with cancer (their late thirties). These are the factors the geneticists base your risks on. So to me, it was kind of inevitable.

I knew that removing my ovaries would be life changing. Giving up the chance of having any more children was heart-breaking. I was weighing up my own risks, thinking about my family, then health, stress, another operation, oh, and menopause . . . that at the time was the least of my worries, maybe because no one talked about it or talked to me about it.

We started to look into the operation . . . but then we accidentally got pregnant with AJ. When I say accident, we all know how babies are made. Anyway, we weren't trying to conceive, but felt that was God's way of saying, "Have another child before it's too late."

When I had the double mastectomy it was obviously before AJ was born – so that meant I couldn't breastfeed. I remember the midwives placing him on my chest as he began rooting for milk. It suddenly hit me that I couldn't feed him. The guilt was immense and consequently I developed postnatal depression. Then, unfortunately when AJ was six weeks old, he had meningitis. As we were in the isolation ward for six days, I began to blame myself because I hadn't breastfed him, which didn't help my state of mind.

I had my total hysterectomy in October 2014, about six months after AJ's birth. We decided on the total hysterectomy over ovary removal after the advice from the medical team. I'd had two c-sections and with that came disruption of the position of the ovaries, so unfortunately keyhole was not an option – therefore they have to cut through, as they would with a c-section. They removed all of the female reproductive organs and, once again, that word came up – "menopause".

I remember thinking, Oh, yes, of course . . . menopause? I suppose, apart from not being able to have children, the only thing I knew about the menopause was my memory of what my mum went through – headaches, insomnia, hot sweats. No one ever really talked about it.

We don't get taught it at school. We don't learn about it in sex education. Yet the menopause happens to every woman and still we are trying to break down the taboo. I'm passionate to change things, to make the next generation of women, Faith being one of them, know it's not shameful, not everyone experiences the same and that it can happen at any age. It's still eye-opening to me how young some of the women I've met have been.

HRT – hormone replacement therapy – again, is something that's not really explained. Not everyone needs it, some can't have it, some women depend on it.

The surgeon who did my hysterectomy put in an implant of oestrogen as I had my hysterectomy. It was implanted into a small incision in my buttock – which slowly releases the hormone over six months – I still to this day have it done. I was so young heading into menopause that my body needed what it was without naturally.

After my surgery, against advice from the doctors, I went back to work live TV presenting for *Lorraine*. It was too soon. I thought I was fine, but I tore the stiches and my scar never fully healed right. I didn't want to let anyone down, let alone Lorraine and her team. If it wasn't for Lorraine Kelly I don't know where I would be. Plus, it was for breast cancer awareness month, something I felt passionately about.

I openly documented our journey on *Lorraine* and with that I was able to interview and meet other women going through menopause, all with their own story and journey. I was meeting professionals, MPs, doctors, all with the same purpose – to educate.

I was struggling in the years to follow. Was I depressed? I don't know. I think that depression can be masking something else. Do I feel like I get depressed? Yes. Is it just hormonal imbalances? Maybe!

Sometimes doctors, no offence, especially male doctors, are a bit scared of the word "menopause". Whether it's through lack of knowledge or ignorance, I've no idea, but I've found it's very difficult to get a man to talk about menopause

One time I went to my local GP. I was struggling with anxiety, insomnia, and I had just slipped a disc in the top of my neck! Taking

Faith and AJ with me, struggling to keep them from wrecking the room, I broke down in tears. I only wanted my repeat prescription of Diazepam to help the pain and, well, help me sleep! As he wrote out the prescription I thought nothing of it, got home, googled the packet and they were antidepressants. I could have taken them. Maybe it could have helped ... I don't know. He didn't explain they were antidepressants and I just know it was a snap judgement for him to give me them without, in my opinion, just cause. Sometimes I imagine my life without early menopause. Sometimes I don't know myself anymore. I'm not myself. I don't feel like me. Sometimes I do, and then I don't. I've always been rather erratic, always high or low, but my highs are not as high, and my lows are way darker.

'Hugh is totally the best husband in the world, but still it's very difficult to talk to those closest to you about something you don't understand yourself.

I don't feel understood — but if you don't understand yourself how can you relay that to anyone? How do I tell my eight- and six-year-old why Mummy is a bit crazy sometimes? Or I'll be extra erratic and then say, sorry. Look, I'm a mum! Sometimes maybe the fact the kids refuse to get out of bed is my trigger, or it'll be the mirror Hugh hasn't put up in six months. Hugh is totally the best husband in the world, but still it's very difficult to talk to those closest to you about something you don't understand yourself.

It's been almost six years now living with menopause. Sometimes when I'm out with friends thinking, Oh s**t, I need to go home. I'm having an anxiety attack and I'm hot-flushing. All while they are talking about life without menopause, usual stuff, kids, husbands not taking the bins out, what to eat, what they just bought online, etc, etc, and I'm thinking, I couldn't get up today for three hours and I hope you can't see my sweat patches.

Look, not every woman suffers the same: 25 per cent of women don't have any symptoms; 50 per cent, like me, have a few, and then there are the 25 per cent who suffer really bad. Some wake up every morning in a pool of sweat or their anxiety is so bad they can't leave the house. We are all different.

The book doesn't stop here. It's been eight years since my reconstruction so within the next year I need to have them redone. The HRT implant now has testosterone with the oestrogen. After about a year of just oestrogen my energy levels, sex drive, my get-up-and-go had all gone. It's helped, a bit, but it's hard to know which way to turn or which HRT is right for you. Lots of people have advice, but it's almost trial and error. I think everyone will have their own menopause journey.

Apart from everything else, my hair is thinner and it doesn't grow. I've also got chin hairs – fun times, LOL. My body is different because the weight distribution has changed. I've noticed that it goes more on my hips and my stomach, which is now always bloated no matter what. Whereas, when I was younger my weight would go from the face down . . . now it goes straight to the middle.

After the double mastectomy and reconstruction, I found I couldn't wear the outfits I used to, as all of a sudden I had boobs that didn't move . . . and you can see the rippling of the tissue and the scars, but hey, I've learned to not give a s**t. I just don't wanna make a statement, so I dress accordingly.

I did a TV interview for *Loose Women* where I revealed my scars. The idea of showing the scars was that it showed confidence within. I remember my manager, Ali, rang me the night before and said, "Don't freak out, but they've asked if you would consider wearing a bikini." I was like, "Oh, Ali, oh God. Oh no. I dunno, I dunno . . ."

I told Hugh, and he said, "Look ... the whole point is that you're trying to say these are your scars, you're proud of them. This is you and people look up to you, so if you can't be confident to show it doesn't matter, then how will they feel?"

I did it and I was shaking. It was the most nerve-wracking thing ever. I was crapping myself! I remember that feeling where you can't catch your breath.

I'm glad I did it. But, in general, I'm hesitant to wear a bikini that is lower than the scars. I mean just because I'm not ashamed it doesn't mean I have to put everything on display. I totally prefer an all-in-one – it's way more flattering and I'm not eighteen anymore.

I am in early menopause because of the decisions that I made. But some women don't have the chance to make the decisions. A lot of women go into early menopause without even realising it, without being correctly diagnosed. There are some who have been perimenopausal for years, and don't seek help because the education still isn't out there and they don't realise what they're going through.

When it all began I kept a diary. I didn't write in it often, sometimes months would go past, but it helped me ... to write down my anger, feelings, thoughts, fears, joys on paper. It was my kind of counselling, which should never be underestimated. With this diary, I was lucky to be able to write my book and with that I was lucky to meet other women, and men, with their own story through either BRCA2 or menopause. There are so many women suffering in different ways, so many. Meeting all of these people along the way, because of the book, has been a form of therapy for me – you all helped because I knew I wasn't alone.

I cry, all the time. I cry a lot and I've been angry. Very angry. Initially the anger was because it was a really difficult decision to make, to go through the operations, knowing I did not have cancer, "just" had a very high risk of getting it.

What my body has been through has been rather traumatic, but I try to not make excuses. I've learned it's okay not to be okay.

I'd say the storm is far from over. It's been a rough year for us all. Covid, consequently the loss of work, being stuck at home looking at the same walls. Hugh working from home, home schooling – don't even get me started! I'd say it's been the toughest time for many of us.

I was angry with the world – for a while – and then I realised everyone has their scars, whether it's physical or mental, on the inside or outside. I've always been a fighter, but to fight the unknown – let's call it menopause – is a battle we haven't won yet. We are only just beginning.

DESIRE

(noun)

A strong wish or want; a sensation of longing,
often sexual. Lust.

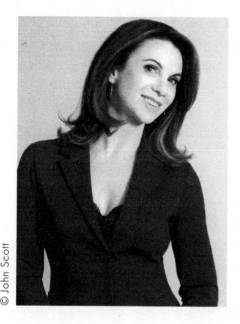

Tracey Cox

Sex expert

"You move on, you change, you experiment, but for some reason with sex we're resistant. Most of us still think sex should look like it did when we were in our twenties. And this is what stops us enjoying sex later in life."

Tracey Cox, 58, is an international sex, body language and relationships expert as well as a TV presenter. She is known for her TV shows on sex and relationships as well as her books, which have sold millions worldwide. She also has her own range of products, developed in the UK with Lovehoney. Her book *Great Sex Starts at 50: How to age-proof your libido* looks at how in midlife and menopause you can still have a vibrant sex life.

~

One of the things I found when I hit the menopause, which shocked me given I'm someone who had such a high sex drive the whole of my life, is that the drive just disappeared. I used to feel spontaneously aroused all the time. I work from home so I would masturbate at least twice a day. And then all of a sudden, I went off sex. I just forgot about it.

It was such a strange thing. Particularly because I'd thought, This isn't going to happen to me. Firstly I'm highly sexed and secondly I know everything. And then all of a sudden it was like, Oh my God, this is no guarantee at all. I'm the same as everybody else. It really has stolen my libido. I have to work at keeping sex alive. It's there, but it's much less spontaneous and that's purely because of hormones.

When my sex drive dropped, it also felt like the nerves in my clitoris went dead. When I researched this, I discovered this really does happen because of the drop in hormones. It's extraordinary how many things hormones influence.

With sex at this stage of life it's almost as if you have to completely rethink it. I'm now oversensitive internally, and undersensitive externally – which is such a weird thing. I never thought this would happen.

Of course, not everyone loses their libido. Part of it relates to the stage of your relationship. I've been with my husband now for eight years and you wonder how much of it is that and how much of it is the menopause. I put myself to the test: the next time I was watching some particularly gorgeous man on Netflix, I asked myself, "If I was single now, if he just presented himself, would I want to shag him senseless?"

My response was, No, I wouldn't actually. I wouldn't because it would hurt.

So it's not just the long-term thing.

There are things you can do to make sex more comfortable. Wearing a buffer helps – it's a squidgy thing that you put on the base of the penis, a thick "love ring", that stops him penetrating too deeply. Changing the way that people thrust is also an excellent idea – keep your pelvises close and grind rather than use the traditional form of thrusting. These things help.

But for most postmenopausal women, including me, desire really does drop. There's no doubt about it. You really have to work to keep it going and sex can hurt, even if you use HRT, even if you are having regular sex.

I was perimenopausal quite early. I reckon I was forty-five when it all started. It coincided with me working crazy hours and I was very stressed, so it was hard to know if it was the perimenopause or all these factors, but I was so angry. I was beyond irritated. I remember seeing my reflection, a glimpse of myself before I'd "arranged" my face, as we tend to do. I thought, Oh my God, look at that angry woman! And then I realised, Oh my God, that's me! I had this whopping great crease in the centre of my forehead.

> "Changing the way that people thrust is also an excellent idea – keep your pelvises close and grind rather than use the traditional form of thrusting. These things help.

I also remember being in a Marks & Spencer's food store, getting groceries and I had about one second to do it in, but I was behind this little old lady walking along and stopping every minute or so and it took all my willpower not to ram that trolley right up the back of her ankles until they were raw and bleeding. I put that in my recent book and my American publishers, who have bought the book said, "Oh no, we can't put that in. That's way too graphic." I thought, Have you never been through menopause? Do you not know the anger that you feel?

Then I got awful hot flushes – just horrible. So I got on HRT which was an absolute blessing and they calmed down. HRT was the magic pill that put everything on an even keel again. I know lots of people can't take it, but I found it was a life-changer.

Something that can make a huge difference to how comfortable sex is – and which I think pretty much anyone can use – are oestrogen pessaries that you insert. Because they are not being taken orally and going through your whole system I think even if you've got breast cancer in your family, you can still take them (though obviously check with your doctor first). They were an instant fix in terms of lubrication.

I know the menopause is different for everyone, but I get annoyed with people who say, "Oh, it's exactly the same after the menopause." It's not exactly the same afterwards for most women and I think we need to stop pretending that it is. Maybe it is for one in a hundred, but for the rest of us it can wreak havoc. I know one woman, who is fifty-nine, for whom I honestly believe it hasn't changed and I know why – it's because she has sex every single day with her partner. I love sex but I'm not sure I'd want that. Would you? Because she has regular penetrative sex, her vagina is probably the same as when she was in her thirties. Sex keeps it elasticised and toned. If you have sex that regularly no matter what happens, you're going to keep your vagina in good nick. It really is "use it or lose it".

What happens generally is most women stop having sex, they get irritated, they have many unpleasant symptoms. Sex falls off, so your vagina is not getting the same exercise. It's like anything in your body; if you don't exercise it, it doesn't work as well. Add things like vaginal dryness and discomfort and hot flushes and you can see why people give up.

And men have the equivalent in erection difficulties, which is a huge deal for them. Women are amazing creatures because we will talk to each other, we're upfront about it, honest and open. Men don't sit around talking about things like we do. They should talk about erection difficulties, but they just don't. ED (erectile dysfunction) is a huge issue for men. It's a psychological catastrophe for men when they can't get an erection. We're dealing with our menopausal stuff;

they're trying to get their head round why their penis isn't working like it did.

This all sounds a bit negative, but I want to be honest. The good news is there is so much you can do. It's all down to attitude. I get that some women who've been married to the same guy for decades get through menopause, sex hurts and they think, Actually, sex is no longer that important to us; we're just going to take it off the agenda. I get that. I know lots of couples who do that.

But if you want to keep having sex – and there's a hell of a lot of reasons why you should – it then becomes all about making an effort and making changes. You have to really put effort into it. But then you have to put effort into anything to keep it interesting long-term. We accept that for most things – but for some reason we resist it with sex. You don't just cook the same meal that you cooked when you're eighteen when you're sixty. You move on, you change, you experiment, but for some reason with sex we're resistant. Most of us still think sex should look like it did when we were in our twenties. And this is what stops us enjoying sex later in life.

We're very resistant to looking at sex as anything other than a bit of foreplay followed by sex based around intercourse. Sex post-menopause should be anything but that. It shouldn't be penetration focused. It shouldn't be orgasm-focused. It should be whatever gets you there. If you can only orgasm now using a vibrator on a high speed then embrace that and do that with your partner.

The problem is there's no realistic portrayal of sex out there. I get so annoyed. I remember in the TV drama *Doctor Foster* they had this scene where you've got this couple who have been married probably fifteen years – more even! – and they just wake up on a Sunday morning and she's, of course, dressed in amazing lingerie that she's worn to bed, and he takes one look at her and next minute they're having mad passionate sex up against the wall.

I watch that and I know that doesn't happen in real life, but even I get a twinge of, "Fuck, that's a bit annoying. Why don't we have that? What's wrong with me?" I know it's not feasible but, even knowing that, it still makes me nervous and like I'm missing out. The sex we see in the media is mythical sex. It's as rare as unicorns. We're constantly being told sex equals frenetic, passionate inter-course. It's never nice, slow, sensual lovemaking. Which is what sex post-fifty can be. It's not the same, it's different. In lots of cases, it's actually better sex for lots of women.

Also let's not obsess over spontaneity. Anticipation is just as good as spontaneity. My partner and I have Sundays sex where we'll plan sex on a Sunday. I've talked about that and people go, "Oh my God, you weirdos." But we like it because that's the only day we get on our own. We go out for a nice lunch, have a few drinks. We take turns and think about what we're going to do. We always do something new. It works for us. That would never have worked for me in the past when I was younger. But I think when you're older it does work. If you don't plan sex in a long-term relationship, it rarely happens. Everything else gets in the way.

Postmenopause is the era for oral sex. It's also definitely, definitely the age for sex toys. And there is a whole generation of women around my age who seem to have missed that whole vibrator thing. Where were they? Anyone who has ever had an orgasm with a vibrator knows how easy it is. Why would you not? They are so effective! If you're oversensitive postmenopause, you can just turn them down; if your nerve endings are less sensitive, you can turn them up. They are a no-brainer for orgasm for women postmeno-pause. If you have lots of oral sex, take the focus off intercourse, use sex toys and talk openly about sex with your partner, sex can still be great postmenopause.

When I was doing interviews for my book, I interviewed lots of women over fifty who said, "Right, I've had my kids, I've done my bit, now it's my time." And leave their partners and find new ones or stay single. Lots of these women are having fantastic sex because sex when you're older in a new relationship is probably even better than sex when you're younger. You're not as hung up on people-pleasing whoever you're sleeping with. Some women are more judgemental about their bodies, but lots are less. This translates well in the bedroom.

Lots of older women are a lot more confident in bed. You know what you want. And at the beginning of relationships desire is so high and all the hormones flood in to make us highly aroused that it overrides a lot of the symptoms of menopause.

So you have two types of women. Some who start a new life and new relationships, who are having great sex, and others in long-term relationships thinking, I've had a lifetime of sex; I can't be bothered keeping it all going. And then the rest of us muddling somewhere in between.

What astonished me was the amount of couples who get on, talk about everything, who are so close, who just stopped having sex, and never talked about it. Never ever. This isn't wise. It's fine to stop having sex, but there does need to be a moment of acknowledgement between the two of you. If there isn't, not having sex becomes the elephant in the room.

I haven't got bored with talking about sex even though I've been doing it for thirty years. It's different now, though. When I was writing my first book, *Hot Sex*, I was thirty, libido out of control. I'd just left my first husband and you can hear the lust in my voice. You can tell when you read the book that I'm really into sex; it leaps off the page.

Now I'm fifty-eight and more relaxed and more (ugh) grown up about it. There's less of that frantic, "I've got to finish writing this so I can go off and have sex myself." It's more: "Okay, so we need to think about this now. We need to take a more considered view."

I identify with women who feel the menopause as a loss. I don't have kids – and that was because I had cervical cancer when I was about thirty. I had two biopsies, which took out most of my cervix. These days it probably wouldn't have been a problem at all because of IVF. Back then the doctors told me, "You're not going to fall naturally pregnant and you'd have to go on fertility drugs." I was like, forget it, I just won't have any kids. Because if ever this was to happen to the right person it was me. I wasn't sure I even wanted kids, to be honest.

Even so, when I realised I was in my menopause, I was a bit sad because it was like, Wow. That really is it now, isn't it? I'll never be able to have a kid now. Not that I'd spent my whole life wanting one. But you don't want that choice taken away even if you didn't want it.

Luckily my husband had a little girl who was eleven when I met her, and is now nineteen, so I have a step-daughter and she and I are very close, so that helped me. It was like, okay, here's a child who I really do love.

I have never been happier than post-fifty. That's partly because that's when I met my partner and I'm in a really, really happy relationship, which helps. Also, I've always been very competitive and ambitious, a perfectionist and a control freak. But something happened after fifty. Maybe because I'm successful enough to think, Just take a breath now. What are you trying to prove? You've already made it. Stop now. Stop trying to kill yourself. Because I was killing myself. I was so stressed with working so hard. I became a little bit kinder to myself, less competitive. I'm probably much nicer now than I was.

I do see HRT as a long-term plan for me – because I'm on a very low dose and I've got none of the contraindications. I do oestrogen gel, probably one pump every other day, and I've just swapped to a progesterone vaginal pessary that you put in once every two nights. Because of my libido drop, I went to have my testosterone levels tested and I found I've got virtually no testosterone anymore. That was a shock because I was tested when I was younger and I had high levels, hence the high sex drive.

The doctor said, "No problem. I'll put you on this testo gel." I used it and within about a week I felt completely different, like my old self, but not in a good way. I remember the first hint that it was working was I was in a spin class and there was this guy next to me, who was about thirty, super fit, and he was going really fast and I nearly gave myself a heart attack trying to keep up with him. I was stuffed if I was going to let him be better than me.

I thought, What is going on? That's the old competitive me. I did get my sex drive back, but it came at a cost. I was incredibly irritable all the time.

Testosterone gels definitely work. But the pay-off – turning back into the "old" me – made it not worth it. But worth a try for other people!

In a way, it's frightening how much we are controlled by hormones. I think I was always aware of that, but menopause makes you ultra-aware of the way your hormones *are* you. When you're younger you're not conscious that a lot of your behaviour is controlled by hormones. But when they drain through the floorboards during menopause you become aware of what they did. You can feel the difference. I knew a lot about testosterone, but I had no idea how the other hormones affect desire.

Sex can be more satisfying as you get older. But straight people, in particular, need to stop thinking of sex as penetration. Make sex more sensual – more touching-based, less expectation. Let yourself be *more* adventurous than you have been. Lots of women get to fifty and think, you know what, I'm actually really curious about what X feels like. I want to try it with my partner and see what that feels like. A lot of women spend most of their lives caring for other people and get to the point where they think, sod it, this is about me now – I'm going to explore my sexuality and I'm going to push myself into new directions that I've never explored before.

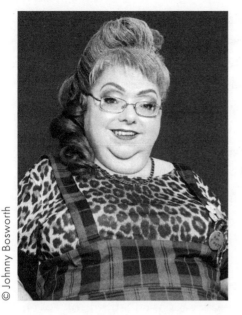

Penny Pepper

Writer and activist

"Punk taught me you were in charge of who you are and what you were doing with your body — and if you wanted it to be grotesque or startling or provocative, you could do that."

Penny Pepper is a writer, poet and activist. Some of her work focuses on disabled people, relationships and sex. She is the author of *Desires Reborn*, a controversial collection of explicit fiction, and she has, throughout her life, rebelled and fought against the spoken and unspoken assumptions towards disabled women. She addresses her experience of the menopause in the same rebellious way. Her approach is outspoken, humorous and political, reflecting the tone of her acclaimed memoir *First in the World Somewhere*.

~

I would say, from my own experience, that the menopause adds to the layers of your medicalisation as a disabled woman. Yet again, you're turned into a medical object. My poem 'Mammogram' (from *Come Home Alive*, Burning Eye Books) describes the experience where I was treated as a piece of meat. And the nurses were women. One was supportive and pleasant, the other one acted as though I wasn't there as a human being. With the menopause it's the same thing. When I was younger I was told I might not even have periods – I have a rare form of arthritis, but, as far as I know, that doesn't involve the womb!

My menopausal symptoms started when I was about fifty-four – so coming up to six years ago. But I was lucky, my mum had a good menopause. When she had a hysterectomy in her forties they left her ovaries – so she would say to me she didn't really notice. My mum is great, not shy or anything like that, and we would always talk about the menopause.

When I first started to experience menopausal symptoms I brought it up with my GP. There was a bit of an attitude of, "Well, there's nothing to be done, that's how it is . . ." I wasn't supported to unravel all the complexities, with my medications and contraindicators. I tried self-help, some alternative remedies since I couldn't be on HRT. Slippery elm, horny goatweed, I took them all to try to regulate my cycle, but also for the emotional swings which formed one of the first symptoms for me.

But I definitely inherited a pattern from my mum in the sense that I didn't have any serious physical issues apart from hot flushes. Out-of-this-world hot flushes. It felt like something had set my body on fire, heat crawling over my skin.

Mostly it was the face – I could have freezing feet and that dreadful feeling of "let me have some air" simultaneously. Sometimes I'd feel like my eyes were sweating. I'm glad to see the back of it. I can cope with my hot flashes – and they're very much flashes – particularly at night. I do everything I can to keep cool – a wet flannel I lay on my face, fan blowing cold – beautiful.

You really don't have any equality in how you're supported in your menopause. Take dryness. I've always had a problem with that because my type of arthritis being inflammatory can give me dry eyes and dry mouth. And if you get dry vagina too, you want to talk to someone about it in a relaxed way. But sometimes, they behave with shock that you're even connected to a vagina.

Looking back, my period faded by blood flow and regularity – and then one day I realised they had gone down to every six weeks. The bleeding was less, and maybe three or four months later I noticed that I'd only have a period for two days. I didn't have a lot of pain. When I was only having a period every eight weeks, I felt happy.

Though I didn't have severe physical symptoms, I did have emotional changes. That was where it hit me. PMT with knobs on, the all-singing all-dancing PMT stuff. Even the horny goatweed couldn't touch that.

While I'm postmenopausal now, I'm still hot – I get the occasional night flush. It's complicated by medication, a vasodilator which can make me burn up too.

I've had a lot of shyness in life. Even getting contraception was nightmarish for me as a disabled woman. I know a lot of women go through similar, and if you add on disability there is that extra level. You have to fight harder to have your menopausal issues heard.

I felt consigned to becoming an old shrivelled prune. Then I thought, So what? I'll be a happy, wise crone. It's part of the experience of life. Women have always struggled to value themselves, confronting the heavy weight of Western culture telling us what to be, how to look and when we lose our value. For disabled women there's another layer, which can be quite contradictory because the cliché tells us disabled women aren't worthy or able to form relationships and bear children, so we fight for that right first and then battle with the right to have a menopause!

I have rebelled against all stereotypes all my life. Sometimes with peer support, and those girls a little older offering insights. I read *Fear of Flying* by Erica Jong as a teenager and it opened my eyes to the reality that women were allowed to enjoy sex. There was also Anaïs Nin's erotica. Somehow, even subconsciously, it dawned on me that there were never any disabled women represented – ever. Not having lovers, not having husbands, not having children. No periods and no menopause!

I feel I have a different perspective and it has been my life's work to fight back against false platitudes. I don't think views have changed as much as they should over the last thirty years – whether we're talking about disabled women having periods, having relationships, having kids (and a lot of women with my condition do have kids), or the menopause. I thought about having children in my late thirties, but as menopause set in I never regretted the ultimate conscious choice I made not to – although it's still exasperating to hear the assumption that it's because I'm disabled.

> One of many positives is that I care much less about what never mattered in the first place.

Most of my friends in my age group are just jealous that I've had the menopause now. We always get support from talking together, emotional strength, realising you're not some weirdo out on the edge coping with this extraordinary thing.

One of many positives is that I care much less about what never mattered in the first place. I feel more relaxed in my own skin than ever before. It's something you hope is going to happen as you get older and for me, it did. I've done nude modelling and burlesque right into my sixties. From my thirties I lost my shyness of getting my kit off because it's a defiant act, and you find out other people enjoy watching you, and that's quite powerful too.

I know a lot of women feel sadness and loss around their body changing and ageing. For me as a disabled woman, I think I've had that journey earlier. I wasn't really going to be shocked at having something else go a bit wobbly.

And I'm a punk in my deepest heart, so psychologically, politically, I've always resisted being on that conveyor belt of what it's supposed to mean to be the embodiment of a biological woman. Punk politics taught me that you don't have to wear a uniform, you don't have to follow a pattern, just because your mum did or your granny. I've got a sharp undercut so when I've got my hair up, I look like I have a cute Mohican. I'm not going to do the cartoon punk, but this is where my feminism exploded. Punk taught me you were in charge of who you are and what you were doing with your body – and if you wanted it to be grotesque or startling or provocative, you could do that.

The menopause has affected my libido, but in a crazy way. I have felt my mojo explode with a sudden binge of, "Let's go on a shag fest, Kevin!" But then other times, I'm like "meh", calm and accepting. I like it because I can enjoy eye candy but it doesn't necessarily connect to the libido in the same way. I rather enjoy being a dirty old woman looking at hot people.

I've always liked writing erotica and I'm working on a novel right now which features a theme around a disabled woman's sexual identity. Disabled women having sex is not a thing you read about and it's time that we did. It needs to be there for other disabled people, it needs to be there as a story, needs to be shown for endless reasons. It's a story from the great, contrary melting pot of humanity. And every human being deserves their place in it.

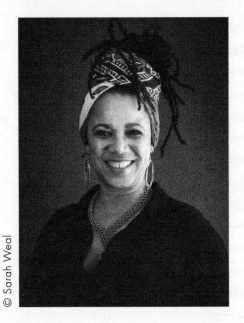

Nimmy March

Actor

"Menopausal sex?
Yes, please. Lots!"

Nimmy March has starred in award-winning television shows including *The Lenny Henry Show*, *Common as Muck*, *40* and *Death in Paradise*. She has appeared in many much-loved soaps and is a prolific voiceover artist. Recently she featured in the online menopause comedy, *Dun Breedin*, a show which she describes as "written from the inside".

~

I'm through it. I had my first child at thirty-eight, my second at thirty-nine, and my third at forty-four. Then, around forty-six to forty-seven, I was perimenopausal. There was a lot going on in those years. I separated from my husband when I was forty-eight, got divorced when I was forty-nine, and I was pretty much done and into the menopause by the time I was fifty-three.

The last years of our relationship were extremely challenging. Splitting was a difficult thing. My kids were ten, nine and five. The menopause was absolutely woven tightly through all of that.

When my periods finally stopped, I thought, Great, it's done with.

I felt a mixture of elation and grief. Because I loved being pregnant, and I absolutely adored the experience of giving birth. I'd had the good fortune to have a friend who was a mixture of philosophical and spiritual in her approach to giving birth. And a thing she had said when she spoke to me about her first birth really stuck in my mind. She talked about how important it was to remember that it was an experience – an interesting experience with a beginning, and a middle and that ultimately it would end. Throughout it, she said, she was always reminding herself of that and choosing to only be in those ninety seconds of extreme contraction.

I really felt like birth is what our bodies are built to do. They are built to do this... and isn't it wonderful to observe the way that our hips open out and everything adapts? It's just amazing. And also, after birth too, I loved finding that my breasts were useful. Breastfeeding felt like one of the best things in the universe to me and I felt very fortunate to be able to do it because it seems that so many struggle.

It's so exciting and it's nature and I love that, actually, we don't really have any control. The only thing we can do is jump on and ride it. I love it because if you're fortunate enough to not need medical intervention then it's the most incredible experience.

Birth for me was magical and otherworldly and extraordinary. And that's where the grief of no longer experiencing pregnancy and having babies again comes from. That was a time in my life, with all three of my children's births, when I felt most powerful. I felt gargantuan and powerful and like I was straddling worlds, straddling the here and now, with the afterlife, with the pre-life, everything.

It felt so massive and extraordinary and I just thought, Fucking hell, women are amazing. It's really incredible to experience your body doing something so natural and so massive that just happens to you. I remember thinking, I didn't ask that muscle to contract and yet there it is.

We spend so much time in the modern world shying away from that which is natural, whether it's with teenagers completely shaving their pubic hair or people making sure that they don't have periods on their wedding day. We're so into using tools and medication to stop our bodies from doing natural things.

Like the whole childbirth thing, the menopause is out of your hands. There's not really anything you can do about it. I remember one of the worst things for me was the insomnia and general sleep issues. And the worst one was being exhausted and not being able to get to sleep, then getting to sleep at two a.m. and waking up at four-thirty. That went on for years and was absolutely exhausting because I'm a single mum with three kids and I had three jobs. So I was wrung dry.

> It was the most amazing and liberating feeling. That perhaps was something that, for me, came with the maturity of the menopause.

I also had very weird and vivid dreams. And there was a lot of catastrophising – a lot of that went on. And weight gain, that was not funny. I've never had a muffin top in my life and there it was. It was like, you must only eat a carrot and you must exercise for twenty-five hours a day and then you might be able to retain some of your former shape.

Another thing that happened is the thinning of hair. I used to have this great, thick hair. The whole loss of pubic hair experience is also not funny. I am not at home to that at all. I've considered a merkin, or maybe a tattoo in a sort of swirly pattern – making it a feature!

It's harder to embrace that lack of control that you get in the menopause than the one you get in childbirth. It's about confirmation of ageing, which is about confirmation of mortality. Perhaps that's what it's partly about – fear of death.

I think one of the struggles of the menopause is that our bodies change a lot, and our brains only mildly. So I think that what's difficult is that you go through this thing which you have no control over. You can control the symptoms by taking drugs or exercise or eating certain foods or whatever, but it's going to happen come what may.

Menopausal sex? Yes, please. Lots! I'm a very sensual person and I enjoy intimacy greatly. I can't imagine not wanting sex, and there wasn't a long period of time in which I didn't want sex during menopause. But it's different for everyone. I'm sure it's different for people who are married, different for women who are married to older men, women married to younger men, and women who aren't married or in an intimate relationship at all.

With sex, of course I like quantity, but quality is the way forward in menopause. Let it be a whole experience rather than just getting down to rutting.

There is a message out there that as a menopausal woman you're going into Crone-Zone, that you are no longer sexually attractive, and unlikely to be sexually active ever again. But that's not what it's like. My body is still horny, my brain is still horny. I still feel very attracted to people.

I've also found new ways of handling new sexual encounters. This all came about because a friend paired me off with one of her friends. She felt she had these two friends who were delicious and gorgeous, both of whom had come out of big relationships, both of whom were not seeking a new relationship, but were seeking sincere affection and intimacy and connection. And she said, "Do you want to meet each other?"

We each said yes and we had a long phone call – and basically that conversation was about coming up with an agreeable contract of how we were going to do this and that it was okay if it didn't work out, but wasn't it lovely that we can get together and have a bottle of wine and a chat. We each committed to taking responsibility for our own emotions. We were clear that "no" meant "no" and "yes" meant "yes" and we reserved the right to change our minds. Because we had our friend in common, we thoroughly trusted each other. It worked so well, and was satisfying on many levels, so we both swore that we would be that upfront and open whenever entering into a new relationship that may involve intimacy – because it was the most amazing and liberating feeling. That perhaps was something that, for me, came with the maturity of the menopause.

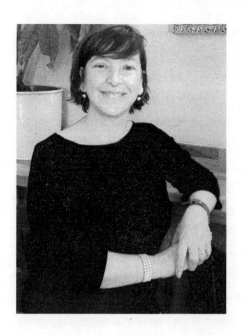

Marie Louise Cochrane

Storyteller

"We're taught badly about sex."

Marie Louise Cochrane, 52, has been a storyteller for over fifteen years and has recently set up Red Velvet Revelry: blog, podcast and live "women's nights celebrating female sexuality – out loud". The end of her marriage, several years ago, led her to throw off repression and explore and talk about her sexuality in new ways. Marie Louise has been a drugs counsellor, Catholic church pastoral worker, healthy food advocate and children's storyteller.

~

I recently started doing storytelling events for women around sex, called Red Velvet Revelry. A few factors made me do this, and one is that, when I came to the end of my marriage, I realised we hadn't been very good at talking about sex at all. We were both Catholics and our cultural formation didn't do either of us any favours in terms of negotiating all that.

I'm perimenopausal at the moment. When I was a teenager, I learned about the Billings method, which allows you to know when you were ovulating by looking at your cervical mucus. So, from right at the beginning, I knew how my body worked and I knew that I didn't ovulate every month. But I had three kids, so obviously I did ovulate enough.

So, I was really aware of how my hormones worked. I even went to see husband-and-wife team, the Doctors Billings, in Melbourne and said, "Do you think I'll have early menopause if I've got poly-cystic ovaries?"

And they said, "You might, so don't hang about if you want kids."

I've always been primed for having an early menopause, but it hasn't happened. I would say, though, that I've been perimenopausal for ten to fifteen years.

A few years ago, while I was still in my marriage, I got very depressed and I thought that was to do with my hormones and the menopause. I got to a point where I got really frightened I was going to hurt somebody. When I was premenstrual, I was really worried I was going to stab somebody in my house. I went to the doctor and they gave me Prozac and I was on it for ten days and I was thinking it wasn't the answer for me. I got a book from the library on cognitive behavioural therapy and that really helped me.

But, looking back, I can see one of the problems was that my marriage was not working and that those kind of homicidal feelings were not my hormones. They were my anger, surfacing when I was premenstrual. So what I thought was an out-of-control menopausal symptom, I now think was something else.

My cycles are now more regular than they have been. I had quite long cycles that were irregular and sometimes I didn't ovulate in the past, but I would say for the last few years they're much more regular. I suspect I'm coming to the end because I'm having big clots.

I've always been quite premenstrual and those are the kind of feelings that are my symptoms – mood swings, waking up in the morning and feeling like everything is terrible (even though nothing has changed), sore breasts . . . my period is probably the same volume of blood but it comes out much more quickly and with lots of clotting, which I never used to have, which breaks through whatever kind of sanitary thing I'm using. It's been so bad some months that it makes me want to stay in the house and not go out.

But I've been using this book by Sally Duffell that tells you how to grow your own HRT, and now I find if I'm taking my red clover sprouts regularly, I can have no symptoms at all. I don't even know I'm getting my period. It's starting to eradicate my symptoms.

More significantly, there has been a new factor in that I'm in a new relationship. I'm wondering if my fertile period has been extended because I'm in a new relationship and having a very active sex life. I think definitely it's shifted somehow. My libido went through the roof. I don't know if there is a hormonal element to that. I know there can be a rise in testosterone at the time of the perimenopause and I don't know if it's that or if it's just being in a new relationship.

The thing about a new relationship is all the stuff that goes with that. At the beginning it was too jaggy. I couldn't sleep. I couldn't eat. Genuinely, it was like being a teenager. Hormonal! Once we got a year in, there was a drop-off for me. It was a relief when the wanting-to-have-sex thing dwindled a bit because it could be frustrating. But it's frightening as well, because it's like, "Oh no, is that it done now? Was it all hormonal or do I really love this person?" I'm happy to say it's all still going very strong!

I noticed that when I was in lockdown my symptoms got worse. I had the worst cramps I've ever had in my life. I had two hours of extreme stomach cramps which I haven't had since I was a teenager. When lockdown started my oxytocin levels fell through the floor – I don't live with my partner, but it wasn't even that I wasn't having any sex, it was that I wasn't having any cuddles from anybody, no physical contact. All of that was affecting my oxytocin levels. My cortisol was up through the roof. I was having to problem solve every single thing I did. I could feel myself on high alert and vigilance.

What was completely different about this new relationship is that, from the get-go, I was talking about the work I was doing with women and sex. We talked about sex right away – and that was partly a test to see if he coped. And he did cope very well! In other words, I was in a completely different space from when I last started a relationship, thirty years ago.

For instance, I was saying I'm a person who feels quite randy when I've got my period. There can be a surge in testosterone around a woman's period. But, in my previous life, that wasn't something that could be talked about. So I said to him, which I couldn't have done in previous relationships, "How do you feel about having sex with a woman who is having her period?"

This was important because I know for some perimenopausal women sometimes it can be ten days, sometimes fourteen, that the period can stretch on for and that can be really inconvenient. I was saying, "That's something I've never been able to negotiate before and I know it's messy, but how do you feel about that?"

And he was fine with it. So that was good. That was really good for our relationship – that I was at the stage where I could talk to him about it, he was able to cope with me talking about it, and we could negotiate it.

"I think I've got some work to do around my sexuality," is what I said when my marriage came to an end and I went to some counselling. Interestingly the counsellor didn't seem very keen to do that, so I ended up seeing a psychosexual therapist. I felt I really wanted to look at it. And now I have.

I'd developed ideas about what pornography meant and its impact – partly through being a drugs counsellor in the 1990s and working with very young women who were given class A drugs to take part. To me it meant exploitation, pain, degradation, antifeminism – I experienced it as something insulting to me. As a result I had never looked at it. So when I became a single person and entered a new phase in my life – where I gave myself permission to explore more areas of my sexuality and make my own decisions about it – I did explore it. I'm not for it exactly, but I can understand that people need and want sexual stimulation. I've worked out that I prefer to explore the life-giving concept of the erotic and separate that from pornography. Audre Lorde's essay on the "Uses of the Erotic" was very helpful for this.

I came to terms with that, processed that. I'd never been in Ann Summers – so I went into Ann Summers and I bought a vibrator. I found out a vibrator is still not a catch-all. My hormones seem to affect not just how I respond to a human being, but how I respond to a vibrator, an inanimate thing. It's not personal – more a case of, I am never going to come, not today, it's not happening.

And I thought, Why can't I go into Ann Summers? Why can't I look at pornography? Why do none of my friends talk about sex? Why is that?

I started to think, Well, I want to be able to talk about it because I talk about everything else. So I created Red Velvet Revelry. I decided I wanted to create a space where women who want to can talk and hear other people's stories and they can hear positive stories. Because everybody can hear nightmare stories. What about the stories that say actually I like sex, actually I still like my husband after twenty years, or actually it's not that great with my husband so I have a sex life of my own. That's what I want to hear about. The live show was created with performer Heidi Docherty, who brings her comic timing and a bit of solidarity – making it easier to talk about this stuff on stage.

I've been thinking back to my fifteen-year-old self. At fifteen I had a good body image. I wasn't doing anything sexually, but I was coming alive and I can see now that that was absolutely petrifying for my parents and they tried to protect me. They told me that men only want one thing. But what I'm actually like is a sexually free and precocious person. All these years I've been slammed into a corner of not even knowing what I'm like and not being able to explore it.

> This is my second half of life. I've been a good girl for my parents. I've been a good girl for the church. I've been a good mother to my children. And now what am I really like? How do I really want to live?

With the confidence of turning fifty, being single, I started looking at, *What beliefs do I want to keep?* This is my second half of life. I've been a good girl for my parents. I've been a good girl for the church. I've been a good mother to my children. And now what am I really like? How do I really want to live? I want to choose what my own values are and not be working out someone else's.

I am always going to be monogamous. I think I'm probably always going to prefer to be with a guy, but I don't rule out the possibility that I could fall in love with a person who happens to be a woman. But I don't really expect that – and I certainly didn't expect to be in love with someone who's twenty years older than me, English, a different social class. But it's his values and his kindness I'm attracted to. So I have to put away some of my prejudices. I've done a lot of work for my business in order to be a more integrated person and this is the next bit of work that needs to be done.

It's been really hard to work out how to market Red Velvet Revelry the right way and not put people off. So I've been focusing on it starting off as a fun night out about sex for women. But what I'm really interested in is deep healing in the area of your sex life and being a whole person and having permission to talk about this in the second half of life and around the menopause. Because if you've never negotiated having sex during your period and now you're a woman who bleeds fourteen days a month, what are you going to do? Who is going to talk to you about that? Your GP isn't going to. There is no Well Woman clinic. There is no peer support for most women. And that's just one aspect.

We're taught badly about sex. There are certain parts of childbirth that are very well attended to and certain parts that are not, and you get to menopause and again you're feeling half the population goes through it and here you are blundering along on your own – making things up or trying to read and make sense of things.

I'm quite into the vulnerability guru, Brené Brown. I think by me taking the risk of telling my stories about sex, and sharing my experience about sex, I am opening a space for other women to do it. I think it's a kind of leadership.

BREEZE

(noun)

A thing that is easy to do or accomplish;
a warm, gentle wind at your back which is
of great help when sailing through.

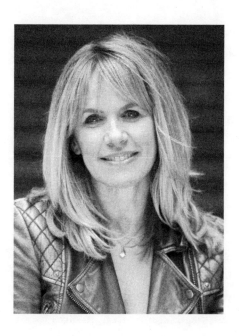

Carol Smillie

Television presenter and
Humanist Celebrant

*"A new door has now opened,
and I'm loving it."*

Carol Smillie, 58, is a former television star who made her name for her appearances on *Wheel of Fortune* in the early 1990s and is probably most famous for presenting BBC's *Changing Rooms*. In the last decade she left television behind and first became an entrepreneur, creating a leak-proof underwear range called Pretty Clever Pants, designed originally for pubescent girls, but later marketed to menopausal women. Then, more recently, she became a Humanist Celebrant.

~

The menopause wasn't a big deal for me. I couldn't pinpoint when my perimenopause started. I knew when your periods stop you've got to go through a year of them not coming back before you're considered menopausal. I didn't feel any grief over the loss of periods – no thanks. But just getting older sucks in general, whether menopausal or not, whether you're male or female. It's not fun. You appreciate your mortality more and think, Gosh, am I becoming invisible?

Looking back, I had a fantastic body when I was younger; but it's not there anymore, well, not in the same way. Let's just say it looks a lot better with clothes on than off! I have two gorgeous daughters, and I look at them and think, *I used to look like that.* And if they borrow things, I laugh and say, "I don't really want it back, thanks very much. It looks far better on you!"

Television is fantastic when television loves you, but there's no knowing when television will fall out of love with you. I had an amazing run. And I think, again, some things are inevitable, and you have to accept them. I had my time and then it passed, and that's fine. For a long time, women over fifty in television were like hen's teeth. You can either choose to fight hard against that, make a lot of noise, and get angry, or you can say, "I'm perfectly capable of trying something else."

That's why I started Pretty Clever Pants, a line of leak-proof underwear for young women – because I thought I could try something completely different, challenge myself, learn a new skill and not be at the whim of someone else. Television is one of the only jobs in the world that you can be really good at, but when you hit a certain age, none of that counts for anything. Those years of experience don't matter, because what matters is what you see. And that's really sad. Don't get me wrong, I'm not moaning about it; it's always been that way and I was certainly happy to take the money when I was younger.

So, for my own self-preservation, I began to look for something else. I started the business because I saw a gap in the market, and the possibilities excited me. It was great to learn something different and be in a whole new world, learning from other people and being my own boss, in charge of my own calendar. But it brought a *lot* of stress too – sleepless nights about finances, stock, customers, education, raising awareness, the list is endless. I started it in 2012, and sold it on in 2018/19, to a TV shopping channel, a bigger player with far more resources, more people and deeper pockets to take it forward. I don't regret a moment of it. I'm very proud of how much I achieved in such a short time.

I'm fifty-eight now. I think the menopause probably started for me at about fifty-two. My mum died nearly twenty years ago, so I couldn't ask her about it all. My older sister hadn't really struggled, she didn't have any great tales of woe, so I just kind of carried on.

There was no particular trigger or point where I thought, *All right, I know what this is*, so I talked to friends about it. Having set up Pretty Clever Pants, our customer profile was originally young girls dealing with heavy periods, but when it was picked up by High Street TV, they marketed it much harder towards the perimenopausal age group, which was really interesting. Firstly, they have more disposable income and secondly, they are more open and matter of fact about body changes. Often, they've been through childbirth, periods, all that stuff, so they totally got what a life-changing product it was.

> This pressure we put on ourselves to have the perfect body on the outside, when it's always been amazing on the inside, is sad.

I always knew that, having designed them for teenage girls, my customers were never teenagers, because they still saw it as Mum's job to pay for something like that. So our customers were mums who recognised the issue for their daughters but would equally buy a pair for themselves, thinking, That's a good idea, I could use that next time I sneeze, cough or someone asks me to go on a trampoline!

Because, with the business, I touched upon that whole market – unwittingly I suppose – I became more educated about the menopause before I reached that stage.

Women's bodies are amazing. We throw a lot at them – whether it's puberty, periods, endometriosis, PCOS, childbirth, stress incontinence, breastfeeding, post-childbirth, or menopause. A LOT of stuff goes on and we need to appreciate that. This pressure we put on ourselves to have the perfect body on the outside, when it's always been amazing on the inside, is sad. We have to learn to love our bodies a little more, warts and all. Social media doesn't help either. Life's not like that, we need to be kinder to ourselves. Men don't put themselves under that pressure. They laugh when they get a tummy, or if they don't look after themselves, they never say, "Did you see the state of Dave? He's really let himself go."

Women worry about their hips / tummy / legs getting bigger, their skin wrinkling, or just getting thicker (another horrible menopause side effect). My body shape has definitely changed, and that just crept up on me.

I'm very lucky in that I'm almost thirty years married to the same guy and he's still my best friend and biggest supporter. He doesn't judge or put any pressure on me whatsoever. He must see it – he's five years younger than me. But his concern would only be if I was unhealthy, and I'm not ... I don't do much sport – in fact, I don't own a pair of trainers (unless you count the platform ones that go so well with wide trousers!). I walk my dogs for an hour a day and shop like an Olympian; those are my sports. I do a wee bit of yoga maybe, but my biggest ally is that I don't drink and I've never smoked. I am lucky in that I have a reasonably good metabolism and have managed to maintain a fairly steady weight – though I've definitely become heavier as the years roll on.

Sometimes you have to accept you are never going to be twenty-one again. So don't try and recreate that look; it's not going to happen. Whatever bit you try and fix, there's another bit waiting and then none of it matches up!

I've had a couple of moments when I've accidentally switched the camera on my phone to selfie mode and thought, *Good grief, who's that?* Before I realise it's ME! We all have bits we hate; for me, it's my neck. I joke that it's like a turkey's wattle, but I'm too scared to do anything about it. I love the winter because I get to wear polo necks, and loads of cosy layers. Clothes can be your friend ... or your enemy. Find your own style, one that flatters *this* stage of your life, and hold your head up high.

I was lucky that I didn't have much in the way of menopause symptoms. I got warm a few times but I didn't break a sweat. It was more like I'd say, "Is it really hot in here?" and everybody would laugh, including me. But I've been so cold my whole life I quite enjoyed it. I didn't wake up in the night with sweats. I had a bit of "duvet-on, duvet-off", but it wasn't bad. I know from women I have met and spoken to there are horror stories about having to change sheets or soaked pyjamas. That's not funny. And it amazes me how long we put up with that before we see anyone about it. There are lots of treatments and ways to control it, but many women don't do anything. If their child was struggling with such debilitating symptoms they'd be right down to that doctor's surgery to sort it. So why don't they do it for themselves?

Possibly I had a little bit of anxiety but I didn't recognise it at the time. I had a couple of moments where I wanted to just burst into tears because I felt someone was being really unreasonable (when they really weren't), but I couldn't make anyone understand. That was a feeling of frustration more than anything else.

I haven't taken HRT, but I do eat very healthily and cook from scratch. I don't know if that's got anything to do with it. I drink virtually no alcohol. I was never a big drinker, but they all joke in my family that I always have an Anadin in my pocket to go with my glass of wine, because by the third sip I'll need it. I've never smoked and I feel like the right weight for me. Possibly these things have had an effect, helping me to have an easier time of it.

I'm now on career no. 3 – or is it no. 4? I have trained to become a Humanist Celebrant with Humanist Society Scotland, so these days I spend my life conducting non-religious weddings, funerals and baby-namings. It's a career that finally values my experience as a public speaker and doesn't judge me on appearance only. It's such a privilege to help people through the best and worst days of their lives, and I'm surrounded by genuinely kind and supportive colleagues. If it's taught me anything, it's that we have one life, so don't waste it worrying about appearance and ageing.

Maybe as I get older, I'm far more philosophical about the madness that I was in for so long and how great it was back then. I look back on those days fondly – and am eternally grateful that social media didn't exist. I have stories, photos and videos to reminisce over, but I don't miss it one bit. I'm a very "cup half full" kinda gal. With each new stage in life comes new opportunities, so why not give them a try? A new door has now opened, and I'm loving it.

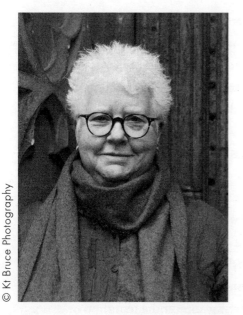

Val McDermid

Author

"I've always been very sanguine about the idea of ageing. I think it's the one war you can't win. It happens."

Val McDermid, 65, is one of the biggest names in crime writing and her books have sold more than 17 million copies worldwide. She grew up in a Scottish mining community and went from there to read English at Oxford. She worked as a journalist for sixteen years before her life as queen of crime kicked off. Val came out as lesbian at nineteen. Her own menopause was far from a big event.

~

The menopause almost passed without me noticing. There was this sudden realisation that I hadn't had a period for three months and I remember thinking, Oh is that it?

It's hard to say when my menopause started because I had quite a long time when I had insanely heavy periods – two super Tampax and a towel would last me twenty minutes sometimes. I had a D&C

[dilation and curettage] in the mid-1980s when I was in my thirties and that helped things for a little while. But they did go back to being pretty constricting in many ways. By that time I was self-employed and I would structure my life around these periods where I felt I couldn't be going off and doing things. I was glad when that started to ease off.

In terms of actual menopausal symptoms, I don't remember having anything particularly disruptive except I did have some strange head sweats. Suddenly, out of nowhere, I would break into a sweat – just my head. My hair would be dripping wet and it would last a few minutes and then stop.

I wouldn't say it was a hot flush, because, from what people have told me that consumes your whole body. It usually happened when I was out and about. I would be buying something in a shop or driving the car and my head would break out into a sweat. It didn't last very long and it didn't happen every day – it didn't even happen every week – but it was the only real physical symptom that I felt that I had.

I've always been very sanguine about the idea of ageing. I think it's the one war you can't win. It happens. So I didn't feel a sense of mourning my young self. Also I didn't have the biological clock thing that so many women speak of and indeed that my partner at the time experienced – this absolute obsession with the idea of motherhood. That obsession of hers was how I came to be a mother, at forty-five, really. But I didn't have that biological imperative at all, so I didn't feel that I'd lost anything.

I came out when I was nineteen and that was the era when you thought, Oh well, that means I'm not going to have kids – that's that. It was one of the things that came with being a dyke back then. You didn't have kids unless you'd had previous relationships with men. So I didn't mourn that particularly. It's a terrible cliché, but

I think for writers, artists and musicians, there's a sense that your work is your posterity – and I never felt the need to replicate myself by having a child. I mean, don't get me wrong, I have loved having a son. It's been a great richness. Though it wasn't something I sought, it was something I embraced.

The one thing about the menopause I definitely felt grateful for was the absence of those periods. Bleeding like a stuck pig once a month was no fun at all. So it was a liberation in many ways. I've seen friends have much more intense experiences – mood swings, flushes, weight fluctuations – but I honestly don't think it's been hugely impactful for me.

My mother had a very difficult menopause. It started quite early, about thirty-eight. She was really ill. She had no energy. She was unwell. She had experienced thyroid issues previously and at this point she kicked into hyperactive thyroid and her weight dropped like a stone. She genuinely had a really tough time. I remember a few years in my teens when my mum was never up in the morning. I'd get up, do my paper round, have breakfast with my dad and I wouldn't see her till I came home from school. That had filled me with some apprehension that when I hit the menopause myself I was suddenly going to lose my energy or my ability to get stuff done. But that didn't happen.

> I don't think I did anything particularly clever to make the menopause easier on me at all. It's just the way it happened and I'm grateful for that.

If anything, I think I've possibly been more productive since I've been postmenopausal than before. I don't feel any slackening of my energies in terms of my creativity.

We had a very interesting experience last year with my partner, who is currently menopausal. We were in New Zealand for two and a half months and after about a month she said, "My menopausal symptoms seem to be so much easier here." She was discussing it with a friend of hers who is a medic and he said, "Have you been drinking the beer?"

Apparently IPA – which is the principal beer in New Zealand – and especially unpasteurised IPA – has a lot of phytoestrogens in it. So there is a strong supposition that it could have a very positive effect on the menopause if you're drinking these particular IPAs that have got strong levels of phytoestrogens. There has been research around their effects, but it has focused on men developing "man boobs". But if they can provoke breasts in men, it's not a giant leap to the notion that they may have a positive effect in menopausal women. So keep drinking the beer! My partner has now discovered non-alcoholic IPAs and that's now a regular feature of our evening meal.

With my own menopause I feel there was a levelling out of my hormones over the month, and I suppose a comparable levelling out of my state of mind. I used to get quite knackered in the days before my period started – I really felt like I was dragging my weary body through the day but I don't really get that anymore. I actually feel that as I'm ageing, I'm healthier and fitter than I was ten years ago. Mostly that's because I made changes in my lifestyle because I didn't want to be falling to bits as I got older. As I say, ageing is the one battle you can't win, but you can try to mitigate it.

I think I dodged a bullet. I got lucky. I don't think I did anything particularly clever to make the menopause easier on me at all. It's just the way it happened and I'm grateful for that.

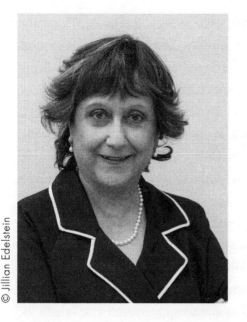

Yasmin Alibhai-Brown

Author and columnist

"After my periods had gone, I missed them. I hated them all those years — and then I missed them."

Yasmin Alibhai-Brown, 70, has written for many major newspapers and she was the first regular columnist of colour on a national newspaper in the UK. She came to the UK in 1972 from Uganda. She is married and has two children, one born to her first marriage which ended in divorce, and the second born when she was forty-three years old. Yasmin campaigns against forced marriages, female genital mutilation, and for the rights of women and girls. Yasmin's latest book is *Ladies Who Punch: Fifty Trailblazing Women Whose Stories You Should Know.*

~

I actually had a relatively easy menopause. There were one or two occasions when I was on television and I was sweating and worried that people could see that. I never took HRT. I never went to the doctor.

I think I was really lucky. I had my second child quite late, when I was forty-three, completely naturally and without IVF or any interventions. Somebody once said to me when you have a child late in life, menopause is less traumatic. I don't know if that's true or not, but that was the case for me. But the thing that did affect me, of course, was mental. After my periods had gone, I missed them. I hated them all those years – and then I missed them. I had a little operation in July 2020 and used a sanitary pad for the first time in a long time. I felt the sorrow of never having to use one anymore. I know it sounds stupid. I actually enjoyed the menstrual cycle. It was the rhythm of life and I used to get very moody during my periods and of course when my first husband used to say, "It's that time of the month," I would get even more angry. But then it was true that I almost unknowingly got more hassled then.

That missing them was mainly because periods are associated with the young side of life for me. And psychologically I felt, Oh my God. It's all downhill from here. For a woman this is it. Nobody wants you. Nobody cares. They just dump you now.

> It was this feeling that I'd crossed a bridge and I'd left behind my womanliness.

I didn't tell anyone I was going through my menopause. I must have gone through it in my late fifties. It was quite late. I wasn't moody, but I did feel grief. That is exactly the word. I felt grief that I had left behind the best part of life. I also feared people's attitudes, so I never spoke about it. But actually I was having a dream menopause. It didn't impact on my work. Except for some moments when I had these hot flushes when I was on television and felt embarrassed – nothing.

It hasn't impacted on my sex life. But I never had any of those problems like vaginal dryness. I am quite lucky to have not had those symptoms.

I did fear in my head that you become invisible, but I didn't feel unattractive. In the end I didn't become invisible, but those were the fears. And it was this feeling that I'd crossed a bridge and I'd left behind my womanliness.

I was on the pill for a very short time. I didn't like the feeling of it. That was the good thing of menopause that we could stop thinking about all that – *contraception*.

I can't, obviously, have another child – but I did have a child at forty-three. We tried for about eighteen months and I had two miscarriages. I'd had a son sixteen years earlier with my first husband and this child was with my second husband. I sometimes think I wish we'd had another when we could have. But, you know, that's just being greedy really.

The other thing is, because with my first marriage, my ex-husband actually left me for a younger woman, there's the fear that men can always do that. I thought, What if this one goes off with someone who is not postmenopausal? In your head you have all these things going on.

Some women, after years of being fed up, leave marriages after the menopause. But I don't think the trend of older men flitting off with young chicks is ever going to stop.

A lot of my friends have suffered during and after menopause. A very close friend physically changed totally and I think she never recovered. She was a very beautiful, slim woman and as she got older she changed completely, unrecognisably – and I think that really does depress her.

For me, though, I was never really known for how I look, but for my brain. Even when I was very young people used to say, "Not a very pretty girl, but a very good brain." So I never felt that was the most important thing about me. I love clothes and I always look after myself and try to look good. It's important to me. I'm like those Black women who whatever age, whatever their class, will always try to look their best. It's a kind of self-love, which we have to keep before and after menopause – particularly after. That was never my big investment in the world – beauty. But I can see if so much is based around that, then physical changes must be hard.

I'm not aware of what my mother's menopause was like because, of course, women in my community and of that generation never talked about their bodies or sexuality or anything. In some ways, by the time they hit forty the women in my mum's circle all behaved old. They were fun to be with. But they thought that was it – they had done their childbearing and now they could be matriarchs. Because actually Asian women love to be sexless matriarchs. It's when they get power.

The mother figure becomes central in the family, perhaps having suffered all their life because there was another matriarch, the mother-in-law; they take that place, oppress the daughter-in-law and they really love it.

I haven't had that matriarch thing going on. I'm too busy enjoying my life and being an independent woman and doing stuff.

Matriarchs can be very anti-female. My mother wasn't like that. My mother was a very lovely and sociable woman. She died about twelve years ago and it was only the last two years of her life that she became dependent on carers – not even that many carers. I took care of her, but it wasn't a huge pressure.

Did I have a midlife crisis? Only about getting older in the world in which I work. I think the BBC, for example, nowadays absolutely never has women over a certain age as presences – and that's just so wrong. We are their loyal viewers! I've been incredibly lucky that I'm still working in the media. I'm still writing a weekly column.

I'm writing other stuff, finishing a book and I get a little bit of broadcasting – not as much as before. Part of it is that I don't think of myself as old. When you stop and you give up and retire, that is when death and old age hang over your head. The longer you can keep working . . . well, it's the way to keep young really.

You have to take care of yourself for health reasons. I do look after myself. I cook every day. I try and get some exercise in. I used to go to the gym – so the Covid lockdown has been quite difficult. I dance to 1960s and '70s CDs in the evening. I slap lots of creams on my face, which I can now afford, but couldn't when I was younger. I do all that.

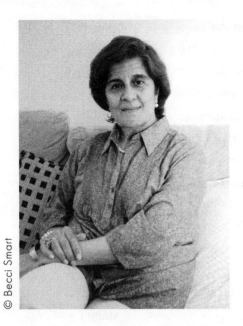

© Becci Smart

Pinky Lilani

Awards founder and
motivational speaker

"The whole thing about being invisible has never been an issue for me because I think I just choose carefully where I am visible."

Pinky Lilani, 66, is a motivational speaker, food expert and women's advocate. She is the founder and chair of the annual Women of the Future Awards and the Asian Women of Achievement Awards. Her midlife has been the busiest phase of her career and in the full flow of all that her menopause arrived, not with a bang, but with a whimper.

~

I may have had a couple of hot flushes but nothing that ever took me to the doctor.

I remember I kept hearing people telling me how rough a time they were having with the menopause or what they were doing with HRT, and I was waiting for mine – but it just didn't seem to come. People were saying it happens in the early fifties, but my periods didn't stop till I was fifty-six or fifty-seven. Suddenly that was it. I thought to myself, Gosh, maybe that was the menopause? It really was a whimper.

I never had any symptoms at all. It was just my periods disappearing and then it was over. It was almost a non-event. I have two amazing sons and two beautiful grand-daughters and I wasn't bothered at all about losing my fertility. I feel this is the circle of life and that's how it comes. I am a Muslim and I think part of that attitude goes back to the spirituality of my religion.

> Sometimes I wonder if maybe my "non-menopause" was because I was so busy.

Sometimes I wonder if maybe my "non-menopause" was because I was so busy. Unlike other people who started working early, the big part of my business, the hard work, started in my forties. At that stage I was very busy doing about three hundred things at once, so I didn't think much about the menopause. I didn't have time. It was only when other people talked about it and discussed these different arguments for and against HRT that I listened. I don't like taking medication, so I was thinking, Would I take it, or would I not? But then I never had to make that decision.

I'm now taking Vitamin D because of the Covid-19 pandemic and that's the first time I've taken any kind of supplement.

However, at the age of forty I started losing my hearing, so I'm actually profoundly deaf and I wear two very powerful hearing aids. I also had Bell's palsy in 2002. Some people recover in six weeks, but it looks like a stroke and that's what a lot of people thought I had. But because I had a highly visible role at the Awards ceremony, I chose not to make a speech but was determined to attend in spite of definitely not looking my best.

So, before my fifties, there were a lot of other things going on with my health that had nothing to do with the menopause. The Bell's palsy was quite a difficult episode but you just have to carry on and, for me, keeping busy is so important.

When people say they want to have Botox or do something to look younger, I've no desire to go down that road. It's really nice to age gracefully, because otherwise you can constantly be having all these nose jobs, cheek jobs, eyebrows, lip fillers done. I have lots of friends who like to look young and who fuss over this wrinkle and that wrinkle. But it's something that I just accept and think, That's life. You can't forever be young.

I did ask my mother about her menopause and hers was also quite late. She said she didn't take any HRT – because her experience was before the time of HRT – and also my mother is one of those people who doesn't make anything of feeling unwell. She just gets on – whereas my father was a bit more of the hypochondriac!

When I was growing up, in India, in a Muslim family, you didn't talk about these things. What we learned about sex and periods was from health science at school. I think now in India they are talking about these issues more, but even twenty years ago it wasn't something you spoke much about. It was something everyone accepted; it came and you just took the symptoms and saw it through.

The whole thing about being invisible has never been an issue for me because I think I just choose carefully where I am visible. I think sometimes you set yourself up for failure. Maybe I was able to choose the right things where, hopefully, I will achieve my goals – though I have had some failures too. You're going to have much more success and a feel-good factor when you're in an area where you can really make a difference.

I didn't feel any dip in energy with the menopause. What drains my energy is when I do things I don't enjoy. Energy comes when you do all those things you enjoy, when you live a life that you feel passionate about.

FREEDOM

(noun)

The power or right to act, speak or think
as one wants; a feeling of liberation.

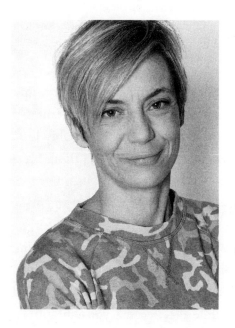

Miranda Sawyer

Journalist and
broadcaster

*"The word care is very
interesting around women and
middle age — because you're
doing a lot of active caring but
you don't care."*

Miranda Sawyer, 53, is a journalist and broadcaster who began her career on *Smash Hits*. She has written for the *Observer* and been a presenter on many television shows including BBC's *The Culture Show*. Ten years ago, after the birth of her second child, she hit what she describes as a midlife crisis, and wrote *Out Of Time*, a moving and perceptive book on the subject.

~

I'm fifty-three now and I first started writing *Out Of Time*, my book about midlife crisis, about ten years ago. My own crisis was triggered by me having my second child quite late, but at the same time I think I was entering perimenopause. I think midlife crisis is started by various factors. It could be a parent dying, it could be losing your job, these sort of things. It's a moment of "Oh my God, where am

I? Is this all there is? I've done it all wrong." That's the common feeling.

The straightforward answer to that question of "Is this it?" is, "Yes, get on with it – that's life." But I don't think there's anything wrong with having a contemplation about where you are. I would also argue, weirdly, that I feel better now, although I probably look worse, and actually I'm in quite a similar situation. And I think I feel better partly because, frankly, I was lucky to have my daughter that late. I also think I was perimenopausal at that time and that can make you feel quite down.

What I've found, in those last ten years, is that I was mourning not just the energy of youth, but also the very strong adrenaline drive I once had. Previously I was living on adrenaline for a lot of my life. There's a dip in that in middle age, because you can't physically carry on doing that really, and you can feel quite low because without adrenaline you just feel like you're chugging along.

It's quite boring and not something you particularly want to get used to. But you have to get used to it, because if you don't get used to it you can't function. The main thing about midlife, which people don't acknowledge, is you're really fucking busy. In your twenties, which is absolutely the time when you should be experimenting, I used to spend days fannying about. Now I never fanny about. I have no days of fannying. It just doesn't happen.

What, anyway, are you going to do even if you do get some spare time? I look at the flat and it's a tip. I've got so much stuff to throw out, as well as all that tedious life admin that you have to do if you're an adult. It's never-ending. So you're always busy, and I'd thought that in middle age you would kind of peak in clutter and somehow you would be sorted and everything would be great – you know, maybe you would have a PA. You would be like the rich women that you imagine or read about. You would just press a button and someone would come round and give you flowers and do your hair and this, that and the other. But that's not the truth for most people. I have come to believe that at no point are you completely sorted out – it's a myth. You just have to organise your head around that really.

It's constant, constant, constant, and if your natural personality is quite teenage, and I think mine is, that's quite hard to deal with. You keep thinking, Oh God, isn't there someone else who should be doing this? The answer is, "No there isn't – it's you."

At this stage, if you've got kids, you're constantly caring. That makes it sound like you're mopping the brow of somebody who is ill. But that's not what caring is. Caring is making sure your kids are where they are meant to be, on time, with sandwiches. I thought caring was being like Florence Nightingale and it's not like that – it's just that you're facilitating the people in your life who need facilitating, and helping so that they can eventually become adults and stand on their own feet. And you do that all the time, nonstop.

I keep thinking I'm in the menopause now. But, annoyingly, I had two very heavy periods right at the beginning of the pandemic. I actually had Covid-19 as well; so, double fun. I was just wiped out. I think the periods you get when you're in perimenopause can be very different. The ones I get are very, very infrequent and really heavy – it's like you're haemorrhaging. When they come, you're like, "Oh my God, what's this? I'm dying. I'd better go to hospital because I've given birth to enormous blood."

I am not yet on HRT. Sometimes I do think about it, especially because it's meant to make you look younger, isn't it? But I'm not used to regulating myself through hormones. I haven't taken the pill for years and years. I've also been in the same relationship for twenty years. Initially, when we were first together, we would do condoms. I did use contraception, but not hormonal contraception. I think that makes me slightly less inclined to take hormones, and so far I've resisted it. I'm certainly not saying I wouldn't: the thing that would push me towards it is low mood. The women I know who have started taking HRT, or been put on Prozac, have done it because of incredibly low mood – that kind of low mood that means not getting out of bed and crying at everything.

What I did have, though, at the beginning of last year, was a period of feeling very flat for about three or four months – just feeling, "This is crap." I wasn't crying at everything or shouting at everybody, which are other symptoms I've heard about; I was just flat. That lasted for about three or four months and then seemed to go away. If that had lasted for a very, very long time, I might have gone to see somebody. But I didn't.

Femininity doesn't really bother me – which is why I dress like a bloke. That's not to say that looks don't worry me, because I think they worry everybody. And actually I went and tried having Botox and fillers for an article in December 2019. I went to this really great woman. I didn't tell her I was doing it for a piece. I thought I could claim the treatments back on expenses, but I couldn't and they were really expensive!

It was very interesting to me how I reacted to having the treatments. Sorry, the tweakments. That's what they're called, *tweakments*. The first thing was no one noticed. Not my husband, not my kids, nobody. But I did and there were aspects of the results that I liked, and aspects of it that really made me question myself. Initially, the first few days, I felt, What is wrong with me? What have I done? I felt like my eyes were too far apart, because she gave me Botox to make the two frown lines in the middle go away. I felt like that had altered the shape of my face. I felt I looked completely different, but, honestly, nobody noticed.

> "What I think happens at this time of life is an adjustment of expectations.

It was a really weird combination of feelings. I felt embarrassed and I didn't tell anybody. I mean, I didn't tell anybody initially, because I wanted to see if anybody noticed, and then I felt, well, I'll have to tell people if I'm going to write about it in a national newspaper. I didn't tell anyone until the feature was about to come out. Then I told my husband, and he was like, "Really? You idiot. Why are you wasting your money?" He was quite funny about it.

I did a picture of before and after, and I looked literally the same, apart from the frown lines had gone and I looked a little bit less tired, which is always what everyone wants to look like. So that was good. *Hooray. Tick. Tick.* And I really liked the woman who did it. But having said all that, I wouldn't do it again.

The whole Botox thing was interesting for me to discover how I felt about myself. I still have vanity. I live in a world where youth is valued, and I look at some photos of me and I think, You look terrible, absolutely awful.

The other thing I noticed about Botox and fillers is – a bit like how after you give birth, you finally know what everyone has been talking about, you join Fight Club, it's the same with this – I can look at the television now and see how everyone, I mean *everyone* on TV, has got Botox and fillers. That was one of the things I found depressing about the whole thing.

I'm worried a bit about aches and pains. I'm kinder to myself than I used to be when it comes to fitness. I think if you walk the dog every day and do a little bit of yoga, that's okay. You don't have to overdo it. I was really into running and I've stopped that partly because I had an Achilles injury ages ago and I was worried about it. Also I can't run with my dog because she just runs off. But there's a trampette class I do and I really love that, and I've got the rowing machine and I've been doing that for twenty minutes every so often during the Covid lockdown. God, it's boring – but I listen to a podcast while I'm doing it.

What I think happens at this time of life is an adjustment of expectations. Midlife crisis is a lot about your expectations. Where did you think you were going to be? What did you think you were going to be doing? All that stuff – you have to make an adjustment around that. It has involved the shrugging off of things I don't really care so much about. Which is good.

You go into midlife crisis and you think, Fuck me, here I am, this is shit. I'm not young anymore, I'm becoming invisible. Though I have to say I don't really care about invisibility, because it's a super-power and it's useful for journalism. But what happens when you get out of that little dip is you think, Right, I've got X amount of time in which to do things.

Whereas men tend to get a divorce at the beginning of midlife crisis, in their early forties, change their wife, get a younger model, I think women when they come out of menopause have a moment and are like, "Right, I'm not going to bother doing *this* anymore, it's boring and pointless."

Caring is interesting when you feel like this. You're still doing the actual physicality of caring, the actual jobs, but you don't *care*. You're thinking, It's fine, I love you and I'm doing this, but I don't *care*. And if you don't like it, I don't care about that either. The word care is very interesting around women and middle age – because you're doing a lot of active caring but you don't care.

A lot of women do get angry in this phase. I wonder if that's related to the not-caring thing. We're in the middle of this weird pandemic, and obviously I could get angry about millions of things, but the problem is that I can't get angry because I'm in the house all the time with my husband and kids. We would have a terrible time.

I'm not bad at controlling my anger. What you don't really want to be is the kind of miffed woman who is constantly pissed off but doesn't say anything. Who's always thinking, *Why am I always the one who has to do this?* It's that thing where you dump the food on the table, in the huff, because you've had to make the meal again. Whereas what you should do is say, "I'm literally the person who hates cooking the most in the house, so somebody else is going to have to do it." Which I have done. My son has to cook once a week or he's not getting his pocket money.

The thing I quite like about middle-aged women is loads of middle-aged women are really chatty. Whereas before you might have slunk off because you're worried about people's reactions, now you don't. I'll chat to everyone – like an old woman. My kids are just like, "Shut up." I'll be like, "No, I want to chat. I want to be part of this community and I don't really care if it's not amusing to you. I'd rather be part of this community where I live."

At the same time as I was going through the perimenopause, my kids were very small and I was experiencing that slight loss of sense of self that comes with caring for small children. That loss of sense of self, generally, when you have a kid is just devastating, and you have to work through it. Maybe some people don't find it devastating, but for most of the people I know, who are working women, it's completely devastating. You're like, "Who am I? I'm just someone who provides for this thing – and I love this thing, this beautiful baby. But who am I?"

You feel like you're in a cage and you can't leave and you can't be spontaneous. Then as you get older, there are difficulties around having older kids – maybe you have to take up cudgels for them at school. But it's a different thing and also you can see the time when they're going to be gone. My son's fourteen – he's out the door in four years.

I'm less individualistic now than I used to be. Perhaps you wake up a bit. Without even really meaning to, you believed the capitalist dream, but now you start thinking, Actually, that doesn't really work. Lots of money would be great, but you know it's not going to satisfy the hole in your soul. It's not going to make things better for anyone else. I do think there is an element of learning those things that can lead women to be less – in inverted commas – caring.

I like being physically invisible – because then you can make yourself uninvisible. People feel like they're not visible because they don't feel sexually attractive and they don't get shouted at by idiot blokes – whereas I say, "This is great!" I'm completely happy that nobody is shouting at me in the street. What it means is that you can move with relative anonymity through the world, which I find quite useful and then, if I want to be unanonymous, I will talk and I will no longer be anonymous. That's fine.

I'm desperate for my periods to end. I really want to be out the other side. I'm bored of it. I keep throwing away all my tampons in joy, then it fucking comes back again. I'm very happy not to be fertile. I don't want any more children. I imagine I would feel differently if I hadn't had kids. But no, I couldn't give a shit about lack of fertility. There's a freedom to this next stage, isn't there? Fertility is a funny thing because you spend all those years trying not to get pregnant, then you spend years trying to get pregnant, and then it's all done.

I think how you feel about losing your fertility depends on how much of your identity is wrapped up in whether you're fertile or not, and I suppose the act of getting pregnant and being pregnant is not what I associate with my identity. I associate having children with my identity – but being fertile, I don't care about. There are a lot of people who love being pregnant and it was an interesting process, but it didn't make me feel amazingly womanly. It's just not where my identity is centred, so it doesn't bother me.

Going through pregnancy and having both kids as emergency c-sections was an interesting and valuable and wild experience that I won't have again. But I'll have interesting and valuable and wild experiences that aren't that. I'm very grateful to have gone through it, because it is so life-changing and so amazing. To be taken over by it, to be in that state where your body does all the stuff for you, where you're not in control – that's a very valuable lesson to learn.

The only thing I miss is that there are highs and lows associated with the hormonal cycle, adrenaline and crash, and I quite like those. That's what fuelled me for a long time – emotional highs, emotional lows – and it's what I would miss. I liked having a wild mood and a down mood. I don't want to feel flat all the time, even though I know basically feeling normal all the time means you can get your life sorted out.

What I learned through the midlife crisis is you can get those highs in different ways. You can get it through exercise, you can get it through shagging, you can get it through driving with the window open and playing music really loud, you can get it through dancing – those kind of adrenalised and exciting "life is brilliant" moments can come in different ways. They don't just have to be hormonal.

I don't have an amazing libido at the moment. But I think that's partly because I'm driven by circumstance and I don't find lockdown particularly sexy because I'm not going out and having fun. I suppose it depends what makes you feel sexy and that for me is going out and meeting people.

We still have sex. What you learn in a relationship is that you can feel quite flat, but actually if you start having sex, you'll probably get into it. There was a time when I thought sex was actually getting more painful. But then you just use lube, and that's fine. I assume that was a perimenopausal thing, because I had never really used it before. It must be my vaginal atrophy. Yes. That's... Vaginal. Atrophy.

Sometimes things pass – maybe I was feeling low because the weather was bad. But also sometimes you feel low and then you think, Oh, let's have a crack at it. Just see how you go. I think once you do that, then it's all right really. Basically having more sex and using lube made it better.

People talk about maintenance sex and I do think maintenance sex is quite important in a long-term relationship. It's about accepting it's not going to be fucking brilliant all the time and then just having a shag and then you'll probably feel better about the stuff that was winding you up, like the dishwasher or the bins, or whatever. I know I sound like I'm incredibly pragmatic and unemotional and I'm not – I'm really emotional. But I think when it comes to certain aspects of long-term relationships you should be pragmatic. There are times where you go, "This isn't working, let's try this."

I don't feel any loss of femininity through being menopausal. Also, what is femininity? I am still feminine, because I'm still female. Femininity is a kind of commercialisation or commodification of the idea of being a woman. It's not very interesting. I find more masculine women, and more feminine men, interesting. I don't know why that is. That's just how I am. That doesn't mean my relationship is with a particularly feminine man – he isn't. But I think the people who can question the gender constructs we've been given are more interesting.

When I first wrote *Out Of Time* I was shit scared. There's a metaphor in it about playing a game of chess. At first, you squander most of your pieces carelessly, as if it was some unimportant game, and you say, "Oh can I start again?" And your opponent says, "No. *This* is the game." I used to find that metaphor absolutely terrifying. Now, I think, "Yeah, this *is* the game." I think you have to go through a midlife crisis to understand that – and whether that's associated with the menopause or not, I don't know. It can be for some people – it wasn't for me. It was associated with an identity crisis.

The midlife crisis was originally associated with work, with men having a crisis because they had worked hard but when they hit their middle age, that work success wasn't as satisfying as they thought it would be. That affects women too – it just depends where your identity is located. And, for whatever reason, when I was young I was quite tomboyish and I absorbed the idea of some masculine qualities as being good qualities.

So the menopause has been less of an identity crisis than the actual traditional midlife crisis for me. For instance, I obviously care about ageing. I don't love having grey hair. I've had a clump of grey hair since I was twenty-eight, and now I'm well grey. I'm not so worried about femininity but I am about youth, because no way am I going grey. My crisis is around looking older. But it's still not that much of a crisis. I still don't care quite enough to have a facelift.

Maybe I'm just ahead of my time. Maybe I processed the menopause before it actually hit me. But I think it's to do with the fact I was working in a young industry, writing about young things. I was struggling with losing that adrenaline and potential of youth and asking, "What does that get replaced with?" quite early. Whereas fertility and whether I looked sexy in a bikini, that wasn't bothering me. I now think, Okay, I'm sure I am menopausal. I'm crossing my fingers that I never have another period ever in my life – I don't want them.

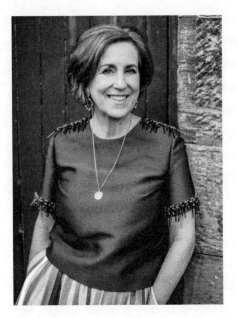

Kirsty Wark

Television presenter

*"We've got to get rid of this
whole idea that you're this dry
old stick and that menopause
is some kind of passage into
a dark world of age and
debilitation."*

Kirsty Wark, 65, is a hugely respected news and current affairs presenter, who has been a key face on BBC's *Newsnight* team since 1993. At the age of forty-six, she had a full hysterectomy and went straight on to HRT. But two years later she stopped it, one of the wave of women who came off the hormones after the Women's Health Initiative (WHI) Study in the United States was abruptly stopped because researchers seemed to have found an increase in breast cancer (and heart disease) with combination HRT. This plunged her into the full range of symptoms.

~

As far as I'm concerned, I've still got elements of my hard menopause. I still get hot flushes and night sweats on occasion and I have problems sleeping sometimes. These are all manifestations of being postmenopausal, but not being quite through it all yet. The point is – that ghastly word – it's a journey. When you're through the menopause I think you need a really big badge, because honestly it's some kind of marathon. It has been for me.

I had a hard menopause because I had a hysterectomy, due to fibroids, at forty-six. The menopause didn't hit at first because I went on HRT, but two years later I came off it, because of the research that emerged then linking it with breast cancer, and I went down with a bang.

I found the lack of sleep quite debilitating. The darkest hour is just before dawn. I would wake up and try and get myself back to sleep by thinking of a wonderful scene in my head. It would be the view over the Holy Isle of Arran from the mainland of Arran, where we would often holiday. What I would often do to get things out of my head is have a notebook and pen – I still do that – and I would write things down. I feel it's only when I write it down, even if it's "buy bread", that it gets it out of my head.

Sometimes I felt sluggish. And that did sometimes affect how I felt about myself, because I then felt the whole of myself to be sluggish. But actually exercise is a massive boost for that because it's an endorphin rush. I was playing lots of tennis, which unfortunately I can't play now. I was doing Pilates.

No one warned me that if I stopped the HRT it would have this impact. I said to the GP, "Look, I'm concerned about the cancer risk." She said, "Well, you can come off it." She didn't explain what was going to happen, though. So I did come off it and I just had to work through it. Now, all these years later, I'm on Vagifem, a much lower dose localised HRT, which helps a little I imagine.

When I had my hysterectomy, I went on HRT immediately, and although the recovery from the hysterectomy was long and sore, I got through it with Volterol and other painkillers. It was those and watching endless series of *The West Wing*, and my family and friends, that got me through my recovery. I didn't feel the effect of the menopause then. I didn't feel it for two years because I was on HRT. It was wonderful.

I came off it at the time of that ridiculous scare and people were talking about it. It was a difficult thing to do. When I stopped, it took a couple of days to hit. I think the first thing that got me was night sweats, and I'm sure short temper as well. Things trigger you.

There's a societal omertà around the menopause. In 2016 I made the documentary *The Menopause and Me* and at that point the BBC had done nothing on the menopause – no documentaries at least. Not only that but, until I came along and said I would tell my story, poor May Miller, the producer, had been on about it for ages to the BBC and they hadn't been interested.

When I look back on that, I'm infuriated by it. I wasn't at all apprehensive about fronting the documentary myself and telling my story. I thought it should be done and I was very happy to do it and bring women's voices to the television. I didn't really care what people thought – if they thought, "Oh she's postmenopausal." I was so far beyond that. I really did not care if there was any adverse reaction – and there wasn't, so it was fine. I thought it was a story that needed to be told, and I felt embarrassed when May came to suggest it to me that I had not thought of it myself.

I feel that documentary was one of the most important things I've done, apart from *Blurred Lines: The New Battle of the Sexes* and some of my big interviews. It was really life affirming. I would have taxi drivers saying to me, "Myself and my wife watched it and it made a big difference to us."

I'm still probably having no more than six hours' sleep. The odd night I have more. I was a much better sleeper when I was younger. This morning I woke up at half six, after not getting to sleep till half

midnight. But then sometimes that's okay. If you're feeling productive then you just get up and do some of your work, perhaps write.
Lots of other people have commitments that mean that if they're
tired it's a huge problem in their day. For us whose work is more
freelance if it's a quiet day you think, Thank God for that.

I don't tend to feel its impact on my working, but what I do feel is
its impact on my wellbeing overall, because of this business of still
having the odd night sweats and hot flushes and not having a great
sleep pattern. What influences my wellbeing more than anything
else is exercise, but because I had a prolapse operation recently I'm
not allowed to run so I can't play tennis to the best of my ability,
which was an exercise I really loved. That is why I need to get my
stamina levels up. I think the fitter you are, probably the easier it is
to cope with.

When I chose to come off HRT, it was a reaction to a friend of
mine who hadn't been very well and had a breast cancer scare. I
should probably not have done it; I should have stayed on it. But
when I was thinking about going back on it again, the doctor said
to me, "You're sixty-two, there's no way. You can have Vagifem
because that's localised, but it's not a good idea to put you back on
it." I wonder what it would have been like to go back on it – but I'm
coming to terms with not actually.

I didn't know Vagifem even existed till I did the documentary
and we looked at different forms of HRT and also what happens to
women's vaginas in the menopause. I remember there was this great
woman who talked about vaginas in the film as all the contributors
sat around my kitchen table.

I very rarely get hot flushes now. I occasionally get them when
I'm flustered about the logistics of travel, when I can't get a booking
or something. That's the time I notice it most. The trouble with the
hot flushes is that they really don't have any rhyme or reason. It

could be a really hot night and you don't get them and it could be a really cold night and you do. It's all internal combustion.

I only had a few occasions when I had trouble with hot flushes on air. But then I asked a couple of colleagues and they said, "No, you looked fine." I chose to believe that!

I try not to take any sugar, which helps, but I can't say I don't take any alcohol. I think when you get hot flushes the only solution is to go away and think about something else, try and read something, look out the window, try and focus on something else. Try and let it go in your head. Of course, that's easy to say especially if you're me and living in a beautiful house in the West End and can look out to trees.

Where am I on this menopause journey? Ultimately oestrogen is draining from your body, and mine must surely be away for ages, because I had a hysterectomy that included having my ovaries taken out. The symptoms are now much less, but they are still there. I'll have a big party when it's all gone.

I took away many things from making that documentary. One was that when I started out I wouldn't have honestly known all the symptoms of the menopause – like aching bones? I was also horrified by how many women had automatically been put on antidepressants. I didn't have that experience, but there were all these women being put on antidepressants by GPs who were recognising that they had the menopause but were saying there was nothing they could do about it, "So we'll put you on these." They had had no talk about the things you can do to alleviate menopausal symptoms. There was no one saying, "We can send you to see somebody, these are the help groups, take a look at Menopause Matters."

For me, I was just so disappointed for women who didn't have any kind of support network and didn't have any way of accessing it – and who didn't even know it was there. And it's only now since the programme that lots of things have happened – like menopause cafés, and also an explosion of companies who are actually actively seeking out speakers to come and talk to their workforces about the menopause.

We've got to get rid of this whole idea that you're this dry old stick and that menopause is some kind of passage into a dark world of age and debilitation. That, in many ways, from medieval times onwards, was how it was seen. I do think there is still a silence. There's that quiet speaking, behind the hand, "She's put on a bit of weight, not doing so well, *menopausal* . . ." We need to get rid of that.

> It's really important for women to talk to their daughters and sons.

My mother didn't speak to me about her menopause when she was going through it. It wasn't until I had my hysterectomy that she said to me, "Oh yes, I had an early menopause." Then, looking back, I realised it had happened at a time of great difficulty in terms of me getting on with Mum. She was forty-six and I was fifteen or sixteen, probably at my most difficult as an adolescent. She could have spoken to me about that but she would never have done. Whereas there's nothing that my daughter Caitlin, and my son James, don't know. It's really important for women to talk to their daughters and sons.

It's interesting if you look out there at the women in powerful positions. Nicola Sturgeon is fifty. Menopausal women are out there really doing things – as are pre-menopausal women, like Jacinda Ardern – there are tonnes of them: Julia Gillard, Christine Lagarde and Dame Jayne-Anne Gadhia.

But also our menopausal years are by and large from forty-eight to fifty-four and that is when women are at the height of their powers, and yet at the same time they're often looking after parents or looking after kids, or both. They're doing everything.

I definitely think the menopause is a liberation. Not having periods is a liberation. But it sounds quite crass for me to say this because I've had kids. I think if you're someone who has had trouble having children, your menopause is probably a terrible flag that goes up to say, "That's it." That must be really hard for people, especially with early menopause.

I also think there's a menopause club. There's a whole load of women who go, "Fuck it, that's it, I can do anything now." Part of it is that we've tried to deal with something and come through it. That's something to celebrate. And if you look at magazines such as *Vogue* and *Harper's*, more and more they include older women in their fashion shoots and features.

As a postmenopausal woman, I've got a new role. As you get older, you just have a different role. You have a lot of things to think about – you've got family, you've got community, you've got work, you've got mentoring, all these things. You've got the idea that you have a certain amount of wisdom that it's good to share.

I would like menopause to be seen as a natural part of our lives. It isn't a choice, it's a natural part of our lives and therefore it should be discussed like every other natural part of our lives. The trouble is, it has been bound up in so much negativity in literature, and it's been the butt of humour. I'm not saying don't be humorous, but let's see who is doing the humour. I'd like fewer men doing menopause humour, more women doing it!

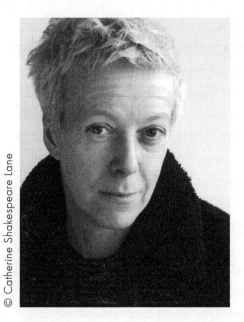

Bunny Cook

Actor

"One of my big problems with the menopause was that I really had to think about female stuff."

Bunny Cook is an actor who uses the pronoun they and identifies as trans nonbinary. They started to experience menopausal symptoms in their early forties, but felt ill-prepared because so much of the information and coverage about the menopause tended to be in the kind of women's magazines or women's health sections of newspapers that Bunny would avoid because they were triggering. Bunny was one of the faces of Holland & Barrett's Me.No.Pause campaign.

~

I'm forty-nine now, and, looking back, with hindsight, I think I was about forty when I started getting symptoms. I still have monthly periods. I hate talking about this stuff, but that is the point of the conversation. My periods vary a lot now – that was one of the signs for me that something was changing. They used to be bang on every four weeks and not really a problem, which was brilliant because, from my point of view, I didn't have to think about it. And then suddenly they started to become more erratic, and much heavier, and then sort of stop and then start again.

What I didn't like was that this stopping and starting was making me think about it and I really didn't want to be thinking about it. I mean, it's great the way we're having this conversation now, but I can only do that because I did the Holland & Barrett ad campaign and all sorts of different talking with all sorts of different people, which enabled me to access that language. But up until that point I hadn't spoken to anybody.

Me.No.Pause was a great campaign – just so innovative in getting lots of media coverage and vocalising lots of different voices. The point I was making in it was that I felt completely excluded; like a lot of people, I realised, once I started talking to the other people in the campaign. Actually a lot of people don't realise their body is starting to have these menopausal changes, because they feel not included. And, as I don't identify as female, I specifically felt not included, and one of my big bugbears – one of the ways I really missed out – is that much of the coverage is often in women's health magazines or those sections of the newspapers. Those are sections that, just for self-preservation, I ignore. So you just don't get those bits of information and I genuinely didn't really understand what was happening.

I hadn't read anything. I think, increasingly over the years, I realised that anything with a female tag was a kind of trigger for me to feel crap, basically. So, I just learned gradually, subconsciously to steer away. I would think, I don't need to know about my fertility levels because that's not relevant to me. So I blocked it all out. My only knowledge of the menopause was that my mum took HRT – and that was to make her happier.

A lot of people have very different experiences, don't they? And it's amazing how, once you start talking about something with people, you then have conversations with all sorts of other people. So because I did the campaign I had a conversation about the menopause with my mum's cousin, which we would never have talked about normally. And she's eighty. She said, "Oh yeah, that happened but I sort of ignored it. It was fine." So, presumably she's either downplaying the whole thing or she genuinely had an easy ride.

I don't really like ticking boxes, but just in terms of helping people's understanding of my gender – that's why we use language, isn't it? – I would say, if I have to write anything down or identify as something, I would say trans nonbinary now. I had chest surgery in October last year, and I genuinely don't think I would have been able to have the confidence or find the way to express that that's what I wanted if I hadn't done the Me.No.Pause ad campaign, if I hadn't had those conversations. I don't know I would have had the confidence to take the steps you need to take to have chest surgery, if I hadn't confronted those subjects. Obviously I'm hugely helped because the world has changed, or at least our little bit of the world has changed.

I don't know when I started to not identify as female, but I certainly never felt female. I had a conversation about chest surgery, back in 1994, a whole other world of awareness, with a surgeon, and they basically wanted to pack me off to a hospital to have a nice little lie down and a few pills. It didn't go well at all. Awful. I was twenty-four, I grew up in rural Cambridgeshire and hadn't read anything about people having gender reassignment. I went to an all-girl school – helpfully. And people would hang around and discuss, saying, "I've got my period." I used to feel awful. I used to feel guilty for not wanting to join in and then they used to kind of go, "Oh Bunny, you know, no need to look embarrassed – it happens to everybody."

I was hugely distressed and didn't want to be playing that part, but, on the other hand, you want to fit in, don't you? They were my friends – I mean I liked all the other conversations that we had.

> It's nothing to do with gender really. It's just physical stuff.

You want to fit in – and all of these feelings stopped me registering that this is what was happening to my body. And actually it's irrelevant that it's to do with gender – it's just a physical change in the way your eyesight changes or you put on weight. It's something that happens and you need to adjust or maybe you need to take something to make it better. It's nothing to do with gender really. It's just physical stuff.

But fitting in was my problem. I would see it in the media or talked about on television, and it was never anybody that I kind of thought, "Oh, you're like me."

I do want to get rid of my periods. I have really wanted rid of them to the point that I basically stopped eating at university for about three or four years, because I wanted that physical change and obviously if you lose a lot of weight then your breasts go, pretty much, and also the periods disappear. So, fantastic – all in one.

How different could that phase have been? That needn't have happened if I knew about queer identity. I also wouldn't have struggled recently, if I had known that the menopause was just something that happened. From my point of view, it wasn't helpful that, in my perception anyway, it was always dressed up as kind of a girl thing. In fact, it was unhelpful.

The first symptoms I noticed were the period changes when I was about fortyish. And mood changes. You just don't know what's going on. You just think, well, obviously, I'm over-tired or being horrible. Why am I being so unkind to my mum? The symptoms were obvious really, but because I didn't want to have that label, because I didn't want to be having anything female, I just kept thinking, Oh I'm obviously stressed about things.

My dad had died a couple years before – and I'd think, The problem is I'm not dealing with that. Or I'd think it was just because of difficulties in my relationship.

I used to get incredibly hot, but not in that sort of hot flush way. I'd just sweat loads and get stupidly hot. I didn't actually look any different really. I would say to people, "Have I gone bright red because I'm boiling?" And they were like, "No, you're fine," which again, didn't help.

Also, it came earlier than I might have expected. There's perhaps a misconception that people maybe are more like forty-nine or fifty – whereas actually it can happen pretty much any time. There's this huge range.

But again I just didn't want to know about it. I didn't want to have an awkward conversation with my GP, who – well, you know doctors can be fantastic, but they generally aren't very helpful especially if you are being a bit vague. And I didn't want to go and have to find out. I didn't want to be googling those subjects.

I didn't talk to anybody. I didn't tell anybody. I think I sort of gradually absorbed bits of information, things filtered through the media, and sometime in my forties I got to the point where I thought, Oh, so that's what's going on.

I did go to my doctor, and said, in a fumbling sort of way, "Can I have some hormone tests?" And they were like, "Well, those aren't very indicative actually, so I don't think we'll bother with those." And then they asked things like, "When was your last period? And how was that different before?" I just didn't want to play, so I sort of closed it down. I thought I would deal with it on my own, and it would sort itself out. But it would have been so much better if I'd been educated by somebody, in a very simple way. I spent a lot of years thinking, Why aren't I coping? What's going on? What's wrong with me? Other people seem to manage fine.

Actually lots of good stuff was happening in my life at the time. I was doing some nice acting work and I'd got a partner and that had been going well for a couple of years – and then didn't. But that happens. There was nothing hugely significant really.

Something that is hopeful is that my new GP is amazing. He was very willing to chat about whether taking testosterone would be helpful for me or whether some kind of HRT, which would have basically levelled out my hormones, would work.

But I'm not on HRT. I don't want to even really talk about it, though I have had those conversations over the last year with doctors about whether it might be helpful to take testosterone, as part of my transitioning, or not. At the moment I've decided not to. I think I'm quite wary because – it's difficult to phrase this without sounding inflammatory – for me that feels invasive. I think it's completely great that other people choose to go down that route, but for me, that feels kind of alien, somehow, and that's not to say that further down the line, I might not try it. I think, also a bit of fear – you don't know what's going to happen.

One of my big problems with the menopause was that I really had to think about female stuff – whereas up to that point I didn't have to at all. I'd buy stuff from Superdrug once every four weeks. And then not think about it, really. I hate even saying the word "period".

It's true that at the end of what's happening is not having to deal with them. That is hopeful. But there's a downside to getting to that other side, isn't there? I've got this foggy brain thing. That's huge.

It was a big concern of mine, about six years ago. I found myself thinking, What's going on? Why can't I read this book? Why can't I remember what I was going to do?

Every four to six weeks, I still get a flurry of female feelings. I feel a lot more female for a few days. It's a weird feeling. I've noticed that, since surgery, during those three or four days of the cycle, I feel like I haven't had surgery. It's a ghost thing. I feel like what was removed is still there. Which for the first few months was quite upsetting, but now I just reassure myself that I did make that big positive change and it's just my body and my brain doing their thing. So there's obviously still something going on, and in those days I just feel much more physically uncomfortable and less sure of myself, kind of a bit like I'm doing some sort of role play. And I look back and kind of think, Oh, that's my school self.

So much of our lives is about our hormones. But there's the issue of how much society genders this. I find a lot of this upsetting. I belong to a running club and they're some of my best mates. But running is gendered. You're measured, put into brackets, you know, thirty to forty or whatever your age brackets are, and it's always gendered. Especially in sport, there isn't a neutral box. So do I mess up their system, and be a bit of a pain?

I don't tend to enter organised running events anymore, because I don't like ticking that female box, or looking for my results on the table seeing that I'm 375th in the female section. It's upsetting and it feels dishonest.

I know a lot of people take testosterone with their HRT. That's one of the things the GP was trying to talk to me about. I'm quite jolly with you now, but I get quite upset with those sorts of conversations and my brain completely kind of nets over, and it stops taking in any information, so I didn't actually understand what he was talking about. He was very nice but then he started saying something about how actually some of the hormones are female and that probably I wouldn't want that. So I just thought, I'll let nature do what it has to do.

We're really thrown a female ideal. I certainly was in the 1980s and early '90s when I was going through puberty and sort of finding my way from school and I think I just knew that that wasn't me.

HRT, for me, is definitely associated with being female. My mum, who has always been brilliantly supportive of me, took it partly because she was pretty miserable. I am wary of it, I suppose because I think that's a thing that women do. So again, I would feel like I wasn't being honest with myself or I was playing a part, if I took that stuff... But it might help, I don't know. I don't really take paracetamol unless I have got a headache that's so bad I can't see straight.

I honestly think I've been through the worst without realising it. I don't get those boiling hot feelings anymore. And I don't, say, get those crazy emotions. It could be that I've just learned to manage it. You see it with toddlers, don't you? Something happens and it spirals and they get wound up and wound up and wound up, and then they realise I'm wound up so they get more wound up. That happens still when you're forty-five. You kind of go, "Oh God, I'm hot. Oh no. I don't like being hot, everybody can see that I'm hot." And you're ten times worse.

The best thing that has happened in recent years is my surgery. I've felt so great, since I had surgery in October, and sort of started going to the barber instead of the hairdresser and having difficult but wobbly conversations about testosterone and being in guys' dressing rooms. So I feel so much better than I did when I wrote that article eighteen months ago, but I think one of the things that's changed for me since the menopause is that I started to turn away a bit from relationships. Because I think it does make me focus much more on my body and my emotions.

A lot of that is to do with me understanding and finding ways of expressing my own gender identity. It has made me think about myself physically and emotionally. That can make you feel quite vulnerable and I think that's made me pull away from some of those closer connections with people.

I do ask myself, "How different would it have been for me if I'd read other stories like mine?" How different would it have been if, when I was struggling at university when I was twenty, I'd known about genderqueer stuff. How different would it have been if I'd been able to think of my body as just a functioning thing that helps me get about, and, you know, every four weeks it throws a little shit at you and then that stops. That it happens to everybody. That it's just a body process.

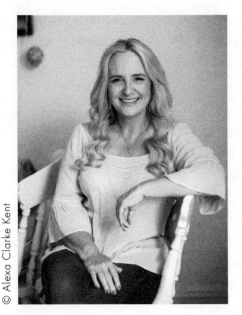

Danusia Malina-Derben

Boardroom consultant

"I would love a rebrand of menopause. I would love it to be around understanding that we are dangerous women. And by dangerous I mean even more powerful than before."

Danusia Malina-Derben, 55, is a boardroom consultant who has maintained a high-powered, multi-decade career, while juggling motherhood. A mother of ten, she'd had four children by the age of twenty-two. When, in her late forties, she had triplets, she found their arrival bumped her into the menopause. Danusia hosts the School For Mothers Podcast.

~

I think the menopause is a journey that really keeps us guessing. There isn't this definitive moment we go, "Aha, I'm in perimenopause." It's just that there is this grey zone. I'm often having this conversations with friends, where we go, "When are we post? When are we pre? What are we?" I feel like we're trying to neatly package this thing called menopause and it isn't neatly packageable.

One of the only ways we know we are perimenopausal is actually going and getting some tests. Then we can say, "Ah, okay, this is where I am." That's how I knew I was in perimenopause. My partner and I wanted to have a last baby – I hasten to add it was a last baby, not a set of babies – and I had tests on my fertility.

Previously, in my very early forties, I had my fertility tested, and they told me then that I had the ovaries of a 32-year-old. I remember they said, "Wow, this is incredible, your store." I like to call it my warehouse. My ovary warehouse had loads of eggs, which was incredible, and knowing that felt really handy. I felt I was younger in that sense. I thought, Okay, that's great; that wins me some time if I ever want more children. I already had seven at this point.

As it happens, I did think I wanted one more and I went, in my late forties, to get my hormones tested again. That time they said, "Well, you are already in perimenopause." When I discovered I had a small amount left, I was like, "Yes, we're going for this!" Because that's the kind of ambitious woman I am!

It turned out I was able to have one more baby. Only that baby turned out to be three. I had triplets. For many women in their mid to late forties, egg donation is the only way. But this wasn't the case for me.

I'm a boardroom consultant. I've had to work really hard, particularly in my early days. And I had my first child at seventeen, so everything has been built with children. Lots of my major clients have no idea I have all these children. Sometimes they'll cotton on and say, "Have you actually got lots of children?"

So I was pregnant in the boardroom with triplets. I was in fairly late perimenopause, on the cusp of the end of my fertility, when I bumped into having these three. I breastfed all of them, which, you know, changes our hormones incredibly. I was in the boardroom while doing that.

It's funny because we have this picture of what a woman with a large family would look like, what her life would look like – she certainly wouldn't be in boardrooms whipping up major PLCs. It amuses me. Of course, it's not amusing work, it's very big, but it just amuses me that we can't have things coexist.

When my triplets were just four months old, when they were barely out of hospital, I had my biggest assignment in my professional life, which was this huge African banking deal.

There's this narrative that when you're menopausal your life will be crunchy and dry and crone-like – but that doesn't have to be the case. I think one of the problems with age and women is that, as a society, we like to categorise the stage at which women are because then we can box them. We can make the right narrative for them. We can say, "Oh, she's drying up; oh, she's not fuckable; oh, she must be knitting."

There's a sea of being labelled or self-labelling that we find ourselves having to push against. We've ingested the shit about what we're supposed to be. All of us are told that we're supposed to be invisible, by the time we're forty-five. What a load of bullshit.

One of the first perimenopausal things I noticed was in my forties I got this libido of a raging eighteen-year-old. I had that rising heat. I've always had a libido for life – and there's a big difference between simply wanting to fuck, and having that wider appetite. My appetite was suddenly big. And that was a bit awkward really, in some ways. I suddenly thought, Oh, what's going on with me? I had an appreciation for what I felt like a boy of sixteen or eighteen might feel like. It certainly wasn't something any other woman around me was expressing – no one.

I'd be on the commute back home and I'd see, for instance, a man opposite roll back his sleeve and I'd just think, *Oof* . . . I didn't do anything but I'd be like, *Oh, yes. Look at that* . . . It just makes me giggle because it was a surge of that feeling.

But when I was with my girlfriends they, you know, they were all moaning or whining about their husbands and not being able to get enough sex, or their husbands being tired, or their husbands bothering them. There was no one who was saying, I am like a little Raging Bull. I kept my mouth shut.

I've read authors Anaïs Nin and Erica Jong and I don't believe any of this is a modern phenomenon. Women for decades have been riding this storm of getting older, learning to be with men if they're heterosexual, having children, menopause, all this stuff, so we can learn from our foremothers. So I learned from some of these authors, and I found, "Actually, I'm not, I'm not that strange."

I had, also, a general rising heat, which was great because I've been extremely cold all my life, so suddenly my temperature was normal. For me, that was nice.

I always say that having the triplets bumped me into the menopause. It was exhausting. I take my hat off to any woman who's attempting to juggle three or four children at once. With three hungry mouths, where do you put them to feed? How to pick three up? It's a whole new type of life because the dynamic of the children is more complex. I breastfed them for at least a year. I would have one on each breast and then, with my foot, I would be balancing a bottle for another one. I mean, I look back and think it was completely mental.

When I say I "bumped" into menopause I mean that their coming was an obvious, discernible moment of change. I can't tell you why, but I knew that something was different, and it's probably because I knew I didn't have that many eggs left.

I haven't felt any mourning around the menopause. My body has been a remarkable instrument and machine for me. Particularly because I worked. We've been to hell and back. We've birthed a stillborn daughter. And I do not take to pregnancy like a duck to water. I don't enjoy it. It's a means to an end. Therefore I'm deeply grateful to her for what she's done for me. But I've done my bit.

One of the good things about having the triplets so late is that it's difficult to feel, "Oh I'm dried up and done" when I've just birthed three children. Or to feel, "Oh, I'm not visible" when I'm pushing a great big long triplet pram. But also I don't feel invisible at all anyway. I am, in so many ways, not done, not a prune, not dried, or any of the awful stereotypes that we get about women who are perimenopausal, menopausal and post.

For a very short while I had HRT but the problem with HRT is I have hemiplegic migraines – though I don't have them at the moment, because actually menopause can be very good for certain types of migraines.

As a child, I started having these migraines when my periods came and they're related to the hormones. I remember my mother saying to the doctor, "So what can we do? Is there a time in Danusia's life when this will end?" The very droll consultant said, "Yes, there is. It's called the menopause." And it is true – it's either pregnancy or the menopause that makes the difference. The kind of paralysing migraines I have are related to hormone patterns.

> I don't feel invisible at all anyway. I am, in so many ways, not done, not a prune, not dried, or any of the awful stereotypes that we get about women who are perimenopausal, menopausal and post.

So, actually, the menopause has been a massive relief for me. But I always knew HRT would not be much of an option. I remember thinking that everything I'd ever read about menopause tells me I'll be invisible, I'll be wrinkly, no one will listen to me anymore, I'll lose all my currency as a human being. And I won't be able to pump anything into me. I won't be able to take HRT.

But then I thought, What's the reality though, Danusia? Are you really any more invisible? Not really. And it's not because I've coloured my hair pink, or changed my physique, or got cosmetic surgery or Botoxed to hell. I haven't done anything. Am I less of a leader? Am I less of a thought leader in my work? Am I less? No.

Have I less of a pep in my step? Have I less energy? Yes, I've got triplets. Fuck, that's hard. They're still young, they're in primary school and I have a special needs child, by the way, quite profoundly special needs. I also left their father when I was pregnant, so I am single by choice.

That's not to say I haven't dated – I've had marriage proposals while I've been menopausal. Life goes on.

I don't feel like the fire has died. In fact, it's increasing. There becomes more of an urgency as we come into our forties. I worried less about what people think of me. Now I don't really give a fuck about what they think of me. And then as we reach the fifties, it's like, oh, I'm changing now. I would love a rebrand of menopause. I would love it to be around understanding that we are dangerous women. And by dangerous I mean even more powerful than before.

I'm a dangerous woman. I'm lethal – in a really powerful good way. I'm not lethal because I'm doing anything awful, but because now I'm on a mission. I'm not as interested in, "Did the men notice me?" Though, by the way, they do. But now it's almost like, "Find someone else. I'm busy. I'm doing my thing."

Have I lost my interest in penis? No. Am I interested in orgasming? Am I interested in pleasure? Am I interested in being a vibrant woman? Yes. That hasn't died. And to those women who say, "I'm dead down there," then I say, "Find your clitoris, find it. Even if you don't have that surge of desire, you have to make friends with that source of yourself."

I believe that centre is our source. That fire is there but it's up to me to stoke her.

My book *Noise: A Manifesto Modernising Motherhood* is published in March 2021. It's a small, mighty book liberating mothers from all that noise telling them who and what they should be. It's a dismantling of what we've been told and tell ourselves about motherhood. The great thing about this is that menopause naturally does it. It dials down the noise. One of the clarities of menopause is that it has us, if we take up the challenge, see what we want.

It has us ask, "What do I want?" For so much of our life, the narrative is about giving our life away to others — our partner, our kids. The bottom line is we only have so much energy, we only have so much time. That's a finite thing. But if we can harness our energy that is the powerful thing.

With the menopause, certainly, if we waste our time and our energy on the narratives around it, then we get pulled down.

An issue I used to have was that I felt my children would eclipse me. I felt people, if they knew about how many children I had, would forget about who I was in my career. But so often our vulnerability is our big strength. The thing we are hiding is often our biggest strength. And it's not that I hid my children — although I did write as an academic about never telling people I had children — but I was promoted and promoted and promoted and nobody knew I had children.

A few years ago I set up School for Mothers, an online community and podcast. One of the reasons I set it up was because I couldn't see anyone else doing it. And I thought, who has got my life experience? I'm occupying an unusual space as a professional woman, not just because I've been working, but because I've been in boardrooms for a long time. For twenty solid years I've been with decision-makers advising them. This places me in a slightly unusual position within those two worlds.

So, when mothers say, "I've never been like this before," I think, Oh my loves. Oh my loves, I can help you.

I have been going through the menopause not just with small children, but also with teens. A lot of women are facing it with teens in their household and that's hard. Literally in their face are these young people's juicy, rampant drive and possibility to get out there and live life, just at the point when everything you read or digest is saying, "You're over. Your husband is going to leave you for a younger woman. You'd better go and get some fillers. You better go on a diet. Go on date night, keep things fresh – otherwise who knows!" All these narratives.

Teens challenge us to find who we are – because they're finding out who they are. And if you don't find out who you are in the midst of teens, God help you. Because you need to have clear boundaries, otherwise they'll gobble you up.

It's at that time, with teens, we have to be sure of ourselves, what we believe, who we are. If you haven't carved out yourself, then it's not suddenly going to appear during their teen years! You will get subsumed under it. I would say that certainly the epicentre of my menopause has been around having teens. There was a time when the triplets were two to three in tantrums, the teens were in tantrums and I was in tantrums. We were all stamping our feet. But we just hung on like it was a rollercoaster ride.

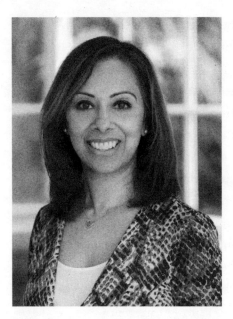

Sharmila Mehta

Immigration lawyer

"The lovely bit about being fifty and upwards is that you don't really care. You don't give a damn."

Sharmila Mehta is a superstar lawyer with more than twenty-two years' experience. She has handled highly sensitive cases around the world, including Russia and the Middle East. When her perimenopause hit, she decided she wanted to handle it naturally and control it through diet.

~

So far, I've been quite lucky in that I haven't really suffered long periods of dramatic change. I had one instance where a couple of years ago, at a Christmas party, I spent virtually the whole evening in the ladies' loos because for some reason my body had just decided that I was going to spend the night bleeding.

Luckily, my friend who is a nurse was there and she said, "Just take some Ibuprofen and it will stop. It will stem the bleeding." And it did. And actually I got to enjoy the last part of the evening. I even managed to get on the dance floor.

I wasn't bothered about the idea of going into the menopause. I felt it was just part of being me and preparing for the next stage in my life. I'm a lawyer and it felt it was coming at the same time as I was making changes to my career. You're not on this rapid ascent anymore. It's more plateauing.

It's been better than I had expected – or had been led to expect from friends, family members and, yes, culture generally. The only thing that's a bit of a bother is the hot flushes. Why is it that they always come on at that particular moment when you're talking to a young man?

I think I've got as much energy as I used to have, but what I don't have is the patience that I used to. But the flipside of that is, I have the expertise, and I know what's going to happen next, because I've been doing it for so long. So, the good part is I'm not as stressed as when I was younger. And the benefit to the client is that you know they've got someone who maybe is a bit more sure about themselves and their advice and won't tolerate nonsense. I'm not pussyfooting around the subject and taking hours. I'll just say, "This is what I think we need to do, and this should be the outcome." The client benefits, but they don't realise they are benefitting.

When I hit my fiftieth birthday, I remember my husband had been saying the year before, "You're going to be fifty soon..." – almost like I should calm down a bit. It was as if he was saying maybe you won't be dancing as much because your knees won't be up to it. Other people seemed to have expectations of what I should look and behave like when I turned fifty. But I just ignored that, and carried on doing what I wanted to, and the lovely bit about being fifty and upwards is that you don't really care. You don't give a damn.

I haven't had anything really to speak of, periods wise, for almost a year now. I think I'm almost in the menopause, though I don't know if some spotting counts as a period. In May, I said to my husband, "Oh, damn, I'm going to have to start over counting that year again. But, hey, you know the upside is at least I'm still fertile. At least I've still got oestrogen."

I have looked up ways to replace oestrogen naturally, because I didn't want to take any tablets. I have upped my soya intake quite a lot, and that makes me feel really powerful, as if I'm in control of my body because I can ingest this amount of soy milk and I reproduce the oestrogen so that I'm having a nice menopause. I'm not sure that's true but I want to believe it.

I want to avoid HRT. I'm a Jain. I'm vegetarian and have never eaten meat and I'm a really non-chemicals person. Also, it does come down again, for me, to control. I want to feel that at this age I really understand my body and I listen to it, and I don't take everything to such an extreme that I need to take artificial chemicals to balance, because this is about balance. And since my grandmothers both lived into their nineties and my mum is eighty, then it seems to me there's something about our diet and the way that we live, that if I can replicate that, then I shouldn't need intervention. I believe the answer should come from nature.

I remember a conversation I had with my GP back in 2018. I went to see him, and I said, "Look, what if I took nothing? What if I just let it run its course?" And he said, "You know that behind this building there is a cemetery. There are enough women who died between forty-five and fifty just from bleeding, because they couldn't control it."

That was such a scary thing to say and actually subsequently I went to see him in 2019, because I'd done some research around bioidenticals. I had heard something on *Woman's Hour* about them and I looked them up and I went to see the doctor and said,

"There are patches that you can get and I want to know about these patches. I want to know about bioidentical hormones." And he said, "I've never heard of those. I've never heard of anything like those patches."

I said, "I absolutely promise you it was on *Woman's Hour*; it's on the internet." Then for about fifteen minutes, he googled it. We sat there and he googled it and nothing came up and he said, "I'm really sorry. I don't know what that is. There's standard HRT."

I felt quite humiliated, the way he did that – that he sat and searched on his computer. I actually sent a letter of complaint to the surgery. I said, "I wasn't making it up. I was made to feel like I was making it up and I wasn't heard. I wasn't listened to." I hadn't named the GP and they wrote back and said, "Would you like to speak to the senior partner?"

I said no, but I think he realised his error.

They did, however, put me in touch with a female doctor and they gave me a priority appointment with her, and I asked every question that I wanted to ask her. More than anything else, she was sympathetic. I didn't walk away with a prescription, because by that time everything was back to normal. I didn't need any help. But it was just nice to know that she was listening. And I wanted to put down a marker – at that surgery and to that GP – that that sort of behaviour just doesn't wash.

> You are not forgotten. You are not hidden. You have wise words and your grandchildren, your great-grandchildren will sit around and listen to your stories.

My family have always been good at talking about body changes. My mum actually would have my cousins over to talk to them because their own mums couldn't. She's very open. We've talked about everything.

It's a kind of conversation I will have easily with all my women friends and family members. Partly I think it's that women stick together in Jainism. You're not allowed to go to the temple when you're having your period and you're not allowed to go to certain festivals when you're having a period. So, it's a community of women where we have the conversation. In a way, having that openness means because it's not a secret there's nothing to be scared of. It's not taboo. It's not hidden. It's nothing to be ashamed of. And it's a natural part of life. It just is.

We have female goddesses and our culture is also quite maternalistic; we're lucky with that. There is this idea that you would be the elder and you would have wisdom and you would be listened to. There is definitely a place for you. You are not forgotten. You are not hidden. You have wise words and your grandchildren, your great-grandchildren will sit around and listen to your stories. There's a real respect for female wisdom and, certainly, older women. They really come into their own.

My work has changed recently. I've moved to a new role in a law firm that is virtual. It feels as if the Covid-19 way of working has followed me. The firm is ground-breaking. It's four hundred lawyers and we all work from home. There is an office and there's a whole structure with admin invoicing people and all of that. But why not have your lawyer working from wherever they want to? Why do they need to be wearing black and white and sitting in a traditional building?

I did it because I wanted that freedom. The freedom and the flexibility to go to the shops in the morning if I want to and deal with my clients at seven p.m. when it's more convenient to them, after they've finished their working day. It was about being modern really, understanding what the future looks like and what young people are looking for. Because, honestly, the thought of going into a dusty old building and seeing a white male in his fifties in a suit and tie and talking to him about your will is dated – and young people just don't want it. I joined the firm just after the Covid-19 lockdown. So it's a really unusual take on life. It was very planned and designed – I didn't want to work in a traditional firm, doing those traditional hours. And frankly, you know, going on the Tube when you are fifty-five or sixty? You just look out of place.

It's been really great for me. I feel I have found my voice. I discovered that I had built a brand. I actually didn't know I had done that. But it turns out I have. And what's good is that I can have my say now. I'm not bound by law firm views and policies. If I want to say that immigration is good for the UK, I can say that. I think that's happened for me at the right time in the world, because people want to hear from those who are in the field, rather than from politicians. We want to look beyond soundbites, to seek the views of experts.

I talk a lot with my daughter, and she used to say to me, "Can I have the old mum back?" She said, "You've become so much more housewife." That was because she was used to seeing that mum, wearing that suit, going into the office, and I must have behaved in a certain way as well. Part of her wants that back, because that was the mum she understood.

My relationship hasn't changed a lot. We've always been very much of a shared mindset. For example, he agreed that I wasn't to go on the pill. He's always been keen to keep things natural, and it's just really very supportive.

I don't think there's enough information out there about the hormones women take. If this was men... if they were taking hormones all their lives, from the age of twenty, this would look completely different. There would be millions of pounds of research into what could happen. There would be different ways of dealing with periods. We would live different lives.

One of the things I object to is this whole thing about women not being allowed to have their hormones fluctuate, and not being allowed to be angry. It's really important to sometimes be angry because you can resolve conflict.

I went to an all-girls school. We were always taught not to be angry. You're supposed to be polite and demure and the rest of it. And I was until I reached sixth form. Our physics teacher, who was quite a strong-willed woman, took six of us to a squash court and said, "I am going to teach you to play squash, because you are going to need to harness that assertiveness. And you can call it aggression, but you will not survive in this world, unless you have it." She taught us to slam the balls. Because we had never, ever been taught that before.

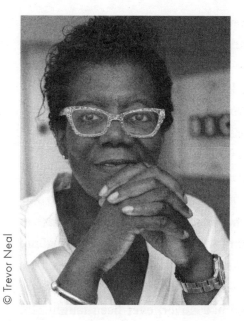

Paulette Edwards

Radio host

"I do believe one of the big problems has been that as a society we haven't talked about these things — whether it's menopause, periods or endometriosis."

Paulette Edwards, 56, is mid-morning presenter on BBC Radio Sheffield. Born to Jamaican parents, she is a former teacher who left the job when she was diagnosed with a life-threatening illness. She started her life in radio running the station's reception. Her menopause didn't arrive with much drama, but after decades of struggling with the pain of endometriosis, a condition in which womb lining grows in places outside the uterus, and infertility problems, the end of her periods brought a mix of feelings. In 2018 she presented a menopause series for BBC Radio.

~

I found a box of tampons the other day and that was weird because I used to have all these tampons and pantyliners in every bag. There was a tinge of sadness, because these were always so much a part of my life. I had extremely heavy periods because of endometriosis and I always had to be ready. I would have paracetamol or ibuprofen, pantyliners, tampons, maybe a few baby wipes, all at the bottom of my bag. And a spare pair of knickers, of course!

It was a bit like going into battle every month. I had the full kit. You also didn't know if you were going to be well for your work. I remember having to be taken home because I was so ill with it.

It's bittersweet when your periods stop and you have had no children because of fertility issues. You're glad that you don't have to be a slave to your periods, because that's what you always were, but then the difficult bit is you're not going to conceive now. I am definitely not going to be a mummy now. There is a balance of those two.

It was difficult to pinpoint when they stopped. I found I'd have a period one month and then wouldn't have them for a few, then I'd have another one. When I realised that probably it had been about ten months, eleven months, and this could be the menopause, I was really sad. Even though I used to have these heavy periods, I wasn't saying, "Farewell and thank God." I was just sad.

I have been quite lucky with the menopause because I haven't had severe symptoms. I've had a bit of being hot. I've had a little bit of being crabby. I've been quite lucky with my sleep, which has been fine. I do remember how when I was doing the afternoon show, at about three o'clock some days, I'd just get hot and then a little bit of heat when I was sleeping, but it wasn't very dramatic. Luckily my sleep hasn't been affected because my sleep's my saviour. I need my sleep.

At fifty-six, somehow, I fell out of periods and there wasn't really a marking point. I couldn't tell you the date that I had the last period. I couldn't really say that and I feel a little bit disappointed because I feel like it should have been a line in the sand. It had been a part of my life since I was ten; it should have been a moment, but instead it phased in and phased out. I was busy. I was just getting on with life. And it was weird because I thought it was going to be monumental.

I didn't even know I had endometriosis until I was about thirty-two. And it was only because of another health problem that I found out. I had fluid on the brain and when I had a shunt fitted to drain it off, I had a full body scan to see if that shunt was working.

At that point they found I'd got a massive cyst on my right ovary and realised that it was due to endometriosis and that I'd got fibroids. I've still got fibroids now. They got rid of the cysts and I had about three or four sets of surgery around the endometriosis.

Before the diagnosis, I'd always had a nightmare with my periods but hadn't realised what that was. I do believe one of the big problems has been that as a society we haven't talked about these things – whether it's menopause, periods, or endometriosis. Not talking about endometriosis has meant a lot of women with endometriosis thought this was just what a period is – vomiting and passing out and bleeding really heavily, suffering intense pain.

A couple of years ago we did a series of shows on the menopause and, after the talk of menopause, the discussion went into periods and a lot of the women were saying that if they had felt more comfortable talking about their periods, maybe the menopause wouldn't have been so much of a challenge.

It's possible my mum had endometriosis too. She used to say that when she used to housekeep in Jamaica – which was really just being a maid – she used to sit on buckets of warm water and that big blobs of blood would come out. It sounds disgusting to talk about, but she said that's the only way she could get her body to relax.

I remember her saying to me, "Sit on this bucket." And I said, "No, I don't want to do it." But then the water was too hot and it scalded me – so that was horrible. It upset her and she never asked me to do it again.

I am comfortable and confident talking about the menopause and other issues now, because I've just talked about it so much. The more I talk about it, the more I think of things as well. I'm quite lucky with friends. I've got about five pockets of friends who I see and we go away, we do things together. We had all these conversations about how it felt for them, what was going on in their head, what was going on in their body, what was going on in their emotions. So the more we talked, the more I thought, if we feel like this, then everyone else must feel like this.

I decided I wanted to cover the menopause on my show. That was partly because every time I met a woman who was my age, all that we talked about was the menopause. But there wasn't any straight-forward information anywhere. You needed to wade through books, and I felt that, anecdotally, it was a lot more useful.

I presented the idea to the editors a couple of times, and they said, "Yeah, it's an all right idea." But then when we had a female editor, who was actually a bit young for the menopause, she said, "Yeah, we do need to do something on this." And we just went for it. It felt like the right time really.

When I was about thirty-three years old, fertility became an issue. I'd just met a fella. I'd just come through the benign cranial hyper-tension treatment, and although I wasn't really in a position yet to try it, I was thinking, Oh, maybe I should try for a baby now.

I was told that if I wanted to conceive, I would have to do it through IVF. But the neurologists thought that wasn't a good idea because the treatment could exacerbate the condition I had with the fluid.

When I decided not to do the IVF, I felt awful, because it wasn't really all my decision – it was partly my body's decision. My mum's got six children, but she had eight pregnancies. She had twins, and she was very fertile – even though there's that chance she could have had endometriosis as well – so I just assumed that one day I would get pregnant, and I wouldn't have to think about it.

I'm not on HRT. And I would have taken it if I'd needed it. I would have, because I suffered so much with the pains of my periods without knowing that I had endometriosis that now if there was anything that was difficult to manage, I'd be quite happy to.

We are all different, and all our hormones are different. I loved it that Jane Garvey said, "Yes, I'm on HRT, because I felt anxious." My friend was the same. She said, "I can't cope with these hot flushes." I think she was having, like, twelve a day, so she said, "I'm going on HRT." Yet another friend who was having twenty-five flushes a day said, "I'm going to try this magnet in my knickers to stop me having hot flushes." She kept losing the magnet. But she said it took her down from twenty-five to twelve when she had it in her knickers. She would forget it was in her knickers and put them in the wash and find it at some point stuck to the inside of the washing machine. Every day there was a magnet story. She was hilarious about that magnet.

I've sometimes wondered if there's a reason my symptoms weren't as *severe*, and it doesn't seem like my mum or my aunties suffered like I know my friends and their mums suffered. My mum was saying the other day that a lot of the food she ate in Jamaica, the traditional Jamaican food, like yam and stuff like that, is stuff that's used to treat menopause symptoms. So I wonder if there's something in that.

There's an attitude in my Jamaican cultural background that, when it comes to the menopause, you just get on with it.

One of the things about the menopause is you're assessing where you are in your life; I suppose you could compare it to the male midlife crisis, although it's a lot more physical for women. It is about assessing what you have done. So for me, I find myself thinking, I haven't got married. I wanted to move house one more time and I haven't been able to do that. I didn't have any children. I love my job – it's the best thing about my life at the moment. I love my family.

The menopause is like a pit stop, where you're saying, "Right, so

337

I've got here. What have I got to show? And where am I going after this?"

I don't think I've had a midlife crisis yet. I think I'm due one. I'm ready for it. Sometimes I think maybe I had it at thirty-two when I was so seriously ill and just thought, Right. So if I've only got five years left or if anything happens, what do I do?

> **I feel quite grateful that I can just focus on myself.**

I remember sitting on the bed when I had the surgery for the shunt and it was pretty full on, and these young nurses came into the room to look after me every morning. I remember one coming in and she had this spiky blonde hair and she sat at the bottom of my bed and she was in such a mess because she drank so much the night before. She said to me, "Paulette, I am so so sorry." And I said, "Don't apologise because you know when I get out of this bed, I want to look like that a few times."

But the menopause doesn't just affect women. It affects men as well. It affects our partnerships. It affects our relationships with our children. I think often we perceive it to be a woman's problem, but it absolutely isn't. It's everyone's issue at work as well, some women not performing as well as they could before.

I feel a bit freer now I'm at this stage of life. I feel really free. And while I would never ever say I'm glad I've not had children, when I look at my friends' lives now, going through the menopause and all the issues that are around with their children, I feel quite grateful that I can just focus on myself. I do feel grateful that if I'm tired, I can be tired. If I'm angry, I'm not necessarily taking it out on anyone else. I can take myself away for a bit and not worry that someone over here can't look after themselves. And so, I think, there's a freedom.

WISDOM

(noun)

The quality of having experience, knowledge and
good judgement, which often comes with age.

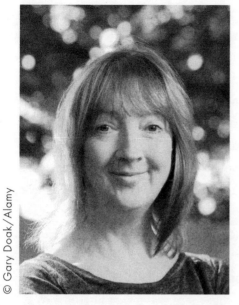

© Gary Doak/Alamy

Sharon Blackie

Writer and psychologist

"Menopause is about going inside. It's really about taking the time to go inside and figure out what on earth this is all for."

Sharon Blackie, 59, is a writer, psychologist and mythologist. In her twenties she worked in corporate jobs, but at age thirty, she had a breakdown, which led to her remaking her life and following her calling. She wrote some of this story in her book, *If Women Rose Rooted*, a rallying cry for a new feminine power. Sharon believes the menopause is an important transition we should embrace and dive into. She is working on a book about elderhood in women, titled *Hagitude*.

~

I had endometriosis most of my life, and the only way of managing it really – and I tried everything – was to be on the pill. But I said to my doctor, "I'm coming off the pill at fifty, because I don't think it's safe after that." I'd kept taking holidays from it all through my life, and decided I would stop it when I got to fifty no matter what happened. I thought I was just going to have to deal with the monthly agony and crippling pain and what have you. So I came off the pill then. And that was it. I never had another period.

That was a really wonderful thing. I'd been dreading the periods because they were so bad. I'd been dreading that sense of them just being unpredictable. So that was a strange one in one way, but it meant that I didn't have the irregularity, and the uncertainty leading up to menopause. Though it didn't mean that I didn't have menopause.

I have described my experience of it as incandescent. I've only become aware of a lot of this with hindsight – I had a lot of life changes at that time, and I wrote my bestselling book, *If Women Rose Rooted*. But I would also say that there was a vast burning away of a lot of stuff I didn't need, and a releasing of issues that I have never been able to get to grips with in my life.

I remember reading Suzanne Moore in the *Guardian*, when she wrote, "I don't really have the mood swings that some talk about. I have just the one mood. Rage." To me it was a little bit like that. It's a stripping away and I think what it does for many of us is it dissolves the boundaries – because it's such an extreme physical and emotional period. I was never allowed to express anger when I was a child and I've always had difficulty in expressing it. That just went out of the window. Now I look back at some of the things that I must have got over-reactive about and think, Oh my God, that was terrible.

I didn't see that maybe I'm just over-reacting to a few things that I had previously tolerated – the shit that I had taken from people, particularly men, all my life! I just thought, *This is great*.

I see the menopause as a very necessary dissolution of some of the things that have held us back. It is an initiation into a new phase of life – whereas we're taught to see it as the end. I mean, come on, it's the beginning. It's wonderful, if you can get through the difficult stages. And every initiation is supposed to be shit. You're supposed to suffer when you go on this initiatory journey, to burn away the dross that opens you up to a new stage in life.

We're taught that it's a failure, it's a dysfunction. But what we're doing is really letting go of an important period in our lives and moving on to another. There's a pattern to life. We had the building phase, the phase which was all about creativity, whether it's in producing children or in other ways, a phase that is about fertility in that kind of very full-on young and middle-aged kind of way, and now it's just shifting that creativity and fertility to another phase of life and we have to let go of all of that old stuff to evolve.

I see menopause as a passage into elderhood. Culturally I think that we've seen it as a loss, a dysfunctional loss of sexuality, a loss of attractiveness and loss of, in some ways, physical health. We also see ageing as a failure, rather than as a natural process of life. We think we have to somehow cling on to youth. But it's a passage – and I think that's why, to me, this idea that we don't go through menopause and that we have to try to medicate ourselves out of it is wrong.

Having done a pharmacology qualification during my neuro-science PhD, I've never taken a drug or any kind of supplement I didn't need to take, ever. But I had to take the pill because of my endometriosis. I started my periods when I was about sixteen, but my endometriosis didn't really come into play until my early twenties. There would be about three or four days out of every month where I was at risk, every minute, of being able to do nothing other than roll around on the floor. And I had a high pain threshold.

My late thirties was the first time that any doctor took it seriously.

I was in America, and a very old doctor said to me, "You shouldn't have had to deal with this all of these years." He said, "What you're going through is the first to middle stages of labour pains every month." That's how debilitating it was. This thing, literally, could come on within thirty minutes, and you wouldn't be able to drive, you wouldn't be able to walk, you wouldn't be able to do anything, so you're going to do what you can to stop it.

When I stopped taking the pill at fifty, I would say the clearest thing I felt, maybe three years on, was I began to realise how very much sharper and focused my thinking was and how – not because of the pill, because that was normalising, but because of hormones more generally – for most of our lives we are completely overrun by emotion. We're driven by that push to mate, whether we think it or not. Had you said that to me in my thirties I'd have rejected you out of hand. I was very intellectual, that was where my focus was, and I would have felt that was bullshit.

But we are overrun by our hormones, and I loved menopause because it took all of that crap away. I felt as if my energy was actually turning to things that mattered. It wasn't that I didn't love my husband; I had a very fine relationship. It wasn't about that. It was just as if a whole burden of cloudy mad stuff had been lifted from me and I had to sit back and think, Okay, now how is this going to work? And that doesn't mean I got it straight away. I think I had a few years where I still overdid it; I still went back to my usual patterns that I wrote about in *If Women Rose Rooted*. But that was such a blessing for me. That this cloudy veil of mugginess had lifted from my head.

I'm not saying that people shouldn't take HRT if they've got particular problems, but I think we have to let ourselves go through a difficult time in order to let the benefits of that later part of life emerge. I think it's such a pity that we don't give ourselves the time and that's part of the problem.

Some women have very serious physical symptoms because of the menopause and have to have treatment to stay sane and healthy, but that doesn't preclude them from doing the deep inner work. It's only when we see medication as an alternative to actually going through the process, or when we take it in order to try to ossify ourselves in this young condition, that it becomes problematic.

Menopause is about going inside. It's really about taking the time to go inside and figure out what on earth this is all for. But our lives don't allow that, and so everybody tries to blunder on through being everything to everybody, the job, the kids, the husband, whatever it might be. They try to carry on as if nothing were happening and take medication to paint over the cracks when really, in any intelligent society, what we ought to have is time for just being.

I was very fortunate because I do work from home. I don't have a full-time job. I don't have kids. And so, even though I didn't realise what was happening, I had the flexibility in the structure of my life to let all of that stuff happen and come out the other side, and most women unfortunately don't.

Of course, it's appealing, the idea that you could not go through something that is difficult. But then that is locking you into an outdated modality. It's stultifying you. It's stopping growth. You've put the brakes on your progression as a human being if you allow that to happen. And, again, it's not individual women's faults; it's the way that society requires us to be constantly productive and that productivity is defined in specific ways by the cultural mythology.

Any good story, any good myth, any good fairy tale will always tell you that the initiatory period when you start on a new journey is going to be tough. But we want everything to be easy. We've lost that understanding that it's supposed to be tough, because in that difficult transition a lot of things get burned away, a lot of things are released and transformed and then you are ready to go into the new phase.

In menopause, we don't really allow time for grieving and I think for anybody it is a time for grieving because you're losing some things that you've been attached to for a long period of time. There's that loss of fertility, sexuality, or attractiveness or whatever, the body changing and wrinkling. It's natural to grieve. But that's part of the process.

If you don't allow that natural grieving to happen, then you can never move on into the next stage of life. And I think that's what we're doing these days in our culture with menopause. We're just cutting it off. We're short-circuiting everything that matters about elderhood, which to me can be very beautiful and very challenging, a very beautiful part of life.

We see it as some failing, as giving in to an inevitable dissolution into death. Of course, it is an inevitable dissolution into death, but that's part of the nature of elderhood.

I had actually done a lot of the things that people do leading up to menopause early. My big life changes were in my early thirties, when I had a breakdown. All of my life, from being a very small child, I had a sense that this was not like a free ride – that I was here to be something, that I had a gift to offer. I didn't really know what it was. I had a difficult childhood, with an alcoholic mother and a violent father. We lived in a lot of poverty; I never really felt safe. Nothing was ever secure. And so I leaped on security, and I took a corporate job that I should never have taken. There was always a part of me that knew it wasn't right. I took it because I needed to pay the bills, because I needed a roof over my head. I didn't quite know what my gift was, but I knew that there was one and this wasn't it.

Whether you're aware of it or not, your unconscious knows perfectly well that the life you are living is completely dissonant, that the persona you are projecting is at complete odds with your whole psyche, and at some point a shift happens. Though I call it a breakdown, it wasn't actually a very acute period, it was just a chronic period of anxiety, a very strong sense of horror at the life that I was living and knowing that was wrong. So that was really what led up to the crisis point.

Then everything after that, my leaving my corporate job, was about finding what it was that I felt I was supposed to be, what I thought my gift was. So really that whole breakdown thing, that whole period, was about a bone-deep knowledge that what I was doing was wrong, absolutely wrong, for me. I was living a life that I actively should not be living.

I think many of us do that in a less acute way. I don't know why I had such a strong feeling from being a child that there was something else to give or do. But I think most of us live with that dissonance in in our world. We adopt personas and have careers and jobs we don't like and we don't see a way out, because life is difficult sometimes and it's not always our fault because society doesn't offer us *options*.

I had to earn a living. I had a mad marriage, which I ran away from, so I had to go back into a corporate environment and go through all of that, again, but it meant that a lot of that reckoning, which many people do in midlife (whatever that is nowadays, let's say in their forties and into their fifties), I did early. So, when menopause came I'd already changed my life, so it was easier for me than it is for many women to go through it. I didn't have the day job where I had to show up looking perfectly groomed and all of the rest of it.

I had also done a lot of work looking back at my childhood, and looking back at the relationship with my mother, and the grief and the abandonment and the wounding and all of that kind of thing. So, to me, building on that journey, menopause wasn't a huge change; it was more a kind of intensification.

In theory, if we lived in a more normal society, by the time people get to late forties and early fifties, which is when the menopause is generally, they should be in a situation where they can afford to take more time for themselves because the kids if they have them will have left home and they don't need as much money because in theory they've got the roof over their heads. But that's not what is happening. Again the cultural mythology is we must always progress, we must always have more, we must always achieve – and so we don't pause.

For me it has been a new journey into elderhood. I've just turned fifty-nine now. Arguably, I began that journey, the menopause, at fifty, a little bit artificially, but the actual menopausal period didn't finish until maybe a year or so ago. So, it's years long, this process for many people, no matter what situation you're in. I think that process of rethinking who you are is a big part of it.

I write a lot about "calling", the old Platonic notion that everybody comes into this world with a gift, something specific to be or to reflect in the world. That's a spiritual belief. I think elderhood is a spiritual passage, and we don't like to talk about those things either. It's too uncomfortable for a lot of people.

I decided that my next book was going to be about the myths and stories of elderhood in women. I really started to think to myself, Okay, so what kind of elderhood am I going to have? What kind of elder do I want to be? And that's a different question. That's a question for this time of life, not for a period of life where I was full of energy and what have you.

That was when I decided to move back to Wales. It was about coming back full circle to the place where my mother moved when I was at university and it always seemed like a secure time. We moved into this house literally a day before lockdown in March 2020. That was difficult, particularly when our movers, having taken all of our stuff from Ireland, refused to deliver them for a month, and we were settling into an old house not knowing how it worked and with nothing to sleep on or to eat or anywhere to sit comfortably.

That stress started up a thyroid condition that had been bubbling under the surface for many years. The main symptom is arthritis – so my hands are a bit buggered. I had that sense of, "So, elderhood isn't necessarily quite what I was expecting it to be." I've had to really take a bit of a dose of my own medicine and slow down drastically. I tend to push pretty hard. I like to do lots of things and this is not a time for that. Menopause should teach us that. I don't think I learned it properly.

This condition that I have means that for the first time in my life I've had to postpone a deadline and say to someone I can't do this book right now, so I'm probably not going to start writing it properly for a while. I've got plenty of pages and proposals and the usual malarkey we have when we produce books. But my whole approach to what I thought was going to be my elderhood has been completely shaken up in the past three months.

I think if we don't do that really intensive deep dive and make the big changes in menopause it catches up with us. For me, elderhood is turning out to be a little different from the way I expected at the beginning, but it is still a gift.

To me, being an elder is about taking everything that you've learned, all the wisdom you've gathered up in your life and then giving it back to the earth and the community. Certainly in Indigenous traditions that's how they would think of an elder. Your time for growing, for building, for accumulating, has stopped now, and you give it back.

I have no role models in my family of what it is to be a good female elder from menopause onwards. All I see, to be honest, are women I don't want to grow into, and that's not their fault either because they didn't have good role models. They were trivialised, they were marginalised; they were told they were silly old women. They were told they didn't have a job and they were just supposed to sit there and watch telly. If you're in the more affluent sections of society, which we were not, you were expected to go play golf or take cruises for the rest of your life.

We're never taught that actually there is something that elderhood represents which is very powerful potentially and very wonderful. I ran a workshop with Pat McCabe who was born a Navajo, and raised in the Lakota tradition, and she told me about the poet and activist Paula Gunn Allen. Her perspective on it is that when you stop bleeding, the blood goes inwards. You're not shedding the blood into the world, so it's available as a creative kind of fiery energy.

There's an inner transformation that makes you capable of putting out a lot of wisdom into the world and a lot of insight and a lot of accumulated knowledge. But we don't have that concept of an elder. The problem is, the community is not receptive. But then, how do you change the community's perspective? By growing really interesting and good female elders who get to do menopause properly and make a proper transition into elderhood. I think it has to start with menopause.

Women are under *incredible pressure* to preserve their inevitably lost youth and look as young as we possibly can. But at some point that becomes untenable. I mean the body just breaks. The body can't do that anymore. Then all of a sudden you're old and you're not prepared for it. You look in the mirror one day and it's like, *shit*. I don't think we prepare for that. Menopause should be a kind of preparation for another way of being in the world.

If you take the classic journey, the initiatory journey, you have the three phases. It begins with the separation from what has been normal up until then, the call to adventure, which to me is the perimenopause. Then you've got the period of initiation, which is menopause itself, and if you want to call it that, the hero's journey (which I don't), the road of trials and what have you, going into the belly of the whale, entering the underworld and all of the difficult shit and the grieving and that dark process which you have to let happen. Then you have the return or "the incorporation" as it's known in anthropology and some Indigenous cultures. I guess, at fifty-nine, I'm on the threshold of some kind of return, or incorporation. I'm getting to the end of that initiatory period, but I'm not quite there yet.

I would say that what I've learned from the whole period of menopause is that it really is, I believe, a time to stop the striving and the building. That's not to say don't do good work. But focus it in. I have a tendency to want to take on all kinds of things. I have too many ideas and I feel this great responsibility to get them out there and to build this and do that. It's now very clear that if I carry on doing that, then in elderhood I will break myself terminally. This whole thyroid arthritis thing is a bit of a wake-up call, letting me know that I still hadn't learned that lesson properly.

But I really do think it's not that you do less work, or you're too tired to do work or whatever, it's just that you focus in on the core of what really it is – Plato would have had this idea of some kind of core gift, some image that you carry around that's like the essence of who you are. Elderhood is a time when all of the other structures that you've built around that start to fade away.

That whole point is that the fiery hot flushes are the classic metaphor for that burning away of all that isn't essential, so that what you're left with is the bare bones of who you are. And that's a really interesting thing and a very beautiful thing to discover. It's that question, "When everything is stripped away from you, what's left? What's there, right at the core of you, when everything is gone, and you can't rely on anything? When everything looks completely fucked, what's left?"

That's what menopause does if we let it, and although that's very distressing and there's a lot of grieving and it's very uncomfortable, what you're left with at the end is this steadily burning flame, which, as I see it, is a beautiful thing. It's different for everybody, but instead of looking at this flame, we tend to medicate ourselves into conformity.

I probably didn't do as much grieving over my changes as some women do. I think it was more of a coming to terms. I find it very freeing. I mean, I've never been a great beauty, but ... Not to be the subject of male attention all the time, not to have that constant self-consciousness – that was wonderful. I like that a lot. So a lot of what many women grieve over, I found to be very liberating. It suited my personality and my sense of privacy and my sense of just wanting to be by myself, with myself.

The only thing I grieved for was all the mistakes I'd made, all the beating up of myself that I'd done over the years, and all of the blaming. I think it's a process also of, at some point, reflecting back on and coming to terms with pretty much every emotional wound you've ever had. That's part of the process and so there's grieving in that. But really it's not grieving in order to think that you failed or that something was wrong; it's part of that process of alchemy, where you shift it then into something more positive, if that makes sense. I'm very much a Jungian in that I believe we have to shift energy, we have to transform it, but we can't transform it unless we really allow ourselves to be in the thick of it.

There was a point where I did want children and I had a bit of a last gasp biological clock ticking. I'd had endometriosis and at that point I wasn't in a relationship, so I decided I wanted to adopt. And then that idea vanished very quickly. I think I'd have been a very bad mother, in that I would have been completely obsessed, and over-responsible for my children, and they would have hated me because of it, and I would have done nothing for myself. I would not have done my work, because I am a born caretaker. I take care of things to excess. I don't see it as a flaw; it's just how it is. So it's probably a good thing that I didn't have children and I don't regret that. Because I think I birthed lots of other things.

I never felt having children was my thing in this life, and I could have easily got diverted and I'm very grateful I didn't. My first husband was much older than me and had a vasectomy in a previous marriage, so that put children out of the question. I don't really do casual relationships and when I met David we were both in our mid-forties so that wasn't going to happen.

I don't really regret that but then you have to, I think, come to terms with what that creative impulse and that fertile impulse during the first half of your life actually resulted in – what was the outlet for it? And what is the outlet for it now, as an older female, which is a very different kind of creativity, I think.

> I've always been very fit and active and that sense of that declining is something I will grieve over considerably rather than any other loss.

I don't mind starting to look older, probably not as much as I ought. It's just going to happen. I don't mean that therefore I'm super enlightened. But this new health issue which has made me think, Okay, I'm going to be cronky now throughout my elderhood, will I never be able to run up a hill again? – that's kind of devastating. I guess I would grieve more for loss of bodily function than I would actual physical looks.

I hope I will still be able to run up hills, because I think I'm just in a flare-up of a condition. But that, to me, is more frightening than wrinkles and sagging bits of this and that. I've always been very fit and active and that sense of that declining is something I will grieve over considerably rather than any other loss.

My next book is going to be called *Hagitude* and it's about the myths and stories of elderhood in women. The word "hag" clearly has lots of connotations that are very negative, but you know in our old stories we have this wonderful archetypal character called the loathly lady. For instance, Kundry, in the story of Parsifal and his quest for the Grail. She comes out of the mist and gives the hero a good shaking and tells him all the ways in which he's completely buggering everything up and how to get a grip. I always loved those characters because I love the idea of a powerful old woman who knows what has to be done to get the world working again.

I like the word hag because it's an acceptance of something that's going to happen to most of us – we're going to get old and things are going to sag. And we're going to be what the world considers to be ugly, but actually many people don't think it's ugly at all. We're going to become in some way hags. But "hagitude" is a bit like hag-with-attitude, it's the idea that we should embrace that, embrace the hagness and what you can do with it. It's not all about being bolshie and noisy and what have you. There is a kind of hagness that is very quiet and very powerful in a different way.

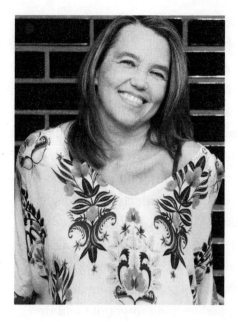

Jody Day

Childlessness campaigner

"The menopause is a huge loss of status to women, and to childless women even more so. Yes, this might all sound quite primitive, but it's still true."

Jody Day is a psychotherapist, the founder of Gateway Women, the global network for involuntarily childless women, and the author of *Living the Life Unexpected: How to Find Hope, Meaning and a Fulfilling Future Without Children*. She was married throughout most of her twenties and thirties and failed to conceive owing to unexplained infertility. After she divorced, she was soon overwhelmed by symptoms – insomnia, anxiety, hot flushes ...

~

Looking back on it, I realise I had my first perimenopausal symptom at thirty-eight, but because it was at the same time as my marriage was breaking down and I was dealing with infertility, divorce and God-knows-what-else, I put it down to stress. I missed my first period that year and then I missed a period each year for the next few years. It was a very stressful time.

That was when my sleep started to change as well – from having previously been a very sound sleeper. It started with waking up earlier than usual and then gradually, over the next few years, progressed to waking up in the night more often, to not being able to get back to sleep, to not being able to get to sleep, to not being able to stay asleep, to basically not being able to sleep at all! It was a gradual collapse of every part of my sleep process over the next few years until it was really critical and I was sleeping only about an hour a night.

I felt like I was losing my mind. The only time I could sleep was in the afternoon, when I would usually get a couple of hours of very deep sleep and that was what stopped me from losing it completely. But as you can imagine, I couldn't do a normal job anymore and so I had to work freelance from home.

By then I was forty-two and, for me, the hideous insomnia was probably the first really big symptom but I still didn't know that it was menopause-related. At that time I wasn't in a stable enough relationship that was suitable to even try IVF in and, after experiencing "unexplained infertility" during my marriage, I was beginning to face up to the looming possibility that motherhood might never happen.

At about forty-three to forty-four, I had my first hot flushes; I didn't know what they were – it never occurred to me that I was in *that* stage. It seemed there were so many things it *could* have been: I was grieving my childlessness (but didn't yet know it was grief); I was depressed; I was really, really struggling with my life, my work, my finances, my relationships, my friendships, my health, my childlessness.

I went to my doctor thinking I had a thyroid issue. She disagreed, but I still ended up seeing this really wacky alternative thyroid specialist for a year or so, who got me taking my temperature every morning; it was like trying to get pregnant all over again. Of course, that didn't do anything – nothing did anything. So I went back to my doctor and she put me on antidepressants. I tried two different ones, but neither of them made any difference – I got the side effects, but no relief from the now crushing anxiety on top of everything else.

There was this moment when it all came to a head for me. I was living in a sweet, sunny little first-floor flat in London which I hardly stepped outside of, I was that ill and anxious. It had a balcony that I more or less lived on and one day the freeholders decided they were going to repaint the building. They scaffolded the exterior and put a green mesh over that and my whole flat was bathed in a gloomy green light and I had noisy, nosy builders on that balcony, able to see right into my space.

It might not sound like much, but that was my limit – the loss of my safe space to hide from the world. I thought, That's it; I'm done – I can't cope anymore. I was absolutely broke but I spent my last pennies on a flight and went to stay with some friends who live in France. My French friend is a psychotherapist and I was starting my training to be one right about that time. She's five years older than me and has female friends ten and fifteen years older than her, all of whom live in the same village.

I remember sitting around the kitchen table with these three women, talking about why I'd had to escape London and how I couldn't cope with anything anymore, and how I would burst into tears at the slightest stress, and they looked at me and said in unison, "You're going through the menopause."

I said, "What?"

They listed the symptoms to me and I was stunned.

"What the hell?!" I said. I was forty-six.

When I returned to London I went back to my doctor again and asked, "Can you test me?" She was a bit reluctant, because of my "young" age, but I insisted. When my results came back she said, "Oh, that was a bit of a brainwave of yours, because you're actually in very advanced perimenopause."

The doctor started talking about HRT, about the risks involved, and I stopped her and said, "Look, right now, I'm calculating the height of tall buildings. Breast cancer is the least of my worries you know, so let's just see how I get on with it."

I started taking the HRT and, within two days, I began to feel more recognisably myself emotionally and cognitively.

I went back two weeks later and the hot flushes had gone – everything had started to normalise. By this time I'd done some research and so I quizzed my doctor a bit more and asked, "How could this have been a 'brainwave'? I'm forty-six: insomnia, weight gain, personality changes, anxiety, hot flushes – all of these things happening? If you don't mind me asking, how much training have you had on the menopause?"

She then told me something which I have since checked out with other GPs and it's true: "Half a day." Half a day! And that was just on the contraindication of prescribing HRT to someone with a family history of breast cancer.

I was stunned. It turns out that in the British medical system, unless GPs have been through the menopause themselves, they are likely to be just as clueless as many of us are because they haven't received any training. This really shows the extraordinary institutional sexism that is still at the core of the medical professional – one which sees women's health problems as less important. Menopause is something that 51 per cent of the population are going to experience – it's not a minor thing! Imagine if doctors only got half a day's training in puberty? It's breathtakingly sexist. And it's cruel.

I was forty-four when I totally accepted that I wasn't going to have children – which was really late – but denial is powerful stuff. Up until then I'd hoped I would meet someone and "do IVF". I was totally ignorant of the likely success rates of IVF at that age; by forty-four it's around two per cent with your own eggs, but because we only ever see the "miracle baby" stories in the media, most people are ignorant of this.

I knew about this thing called "menopause" – I thought it happened to women when they were fifty-one. But I had no idea about the perimenopause, this up to a decade-long process that leads up to it.

I have since learned from a menopause expert that if I had gone to my mother and asked her when she'd completed her menopause, and taken ten years off that, that was probably not far off the time of my last viable egg – ten years before the menopause – that's statistically how it works out. Given, in the end, that I had my last period at forty-eight and was thus postmenopausal at forty-nine, that would have been at around thirty-eight. It's hard to reflect that for so many years I was still hopeful . . . but I was probably already technically infertile.

It would have been absolutely transformative to have understood all this earlier. For example, had I known when my marriage ended at thirty-eight that probably it was game over for me in terms of even *considering* IVF, I would have taken a totally different approach to life after divorce. Most likely I wouldn't have been so focused on finding a new partner to have children with, like right away! I can imagine that I would have headed down a completely different path of self-discovery. I feel like I lost seven years there.

Mind you, they still wouldn't have been an extra seven *easy* years, I'd still have had to face the grief. And finding yourself single and childless in midlife is actually pretty shocking because of the way people view you and treat you as some kind of social pariah. It's a really breathtaking unconscious bias and it's just as strong from women as anyone else. There are some really nasty, very tribal, very painful prejudices against childless women that you don't really see until they're aimed at you.

It's all fuelled by something called pronatalism, which is the patriarchal ideology that dictates that parents are more important than non-parents as human beings, and which functions in a similar way to other prejudices like racism, sexism and ageism. I think it also feeds into attitudes towards the menopause and why we don't talk about it.

The key thing is that once you hit the menopause you're no longer potentially someone's mother. So if you're *not* a mother by that point, you are of no use to the patriarchal project because your usefulness in a very basic biological sense is over and your hormones and looks are signalling that. The only real power you're allowed as a woman in a patriarchal culture, once you're no longer "hot" or potentially fertile, is as someone's mother and grandmother. So if you're neither of those things, you have no acceptable status.

Yes, there are other kinds of "status", but even a high-flying career doesn't make you exempt from the prejudice against childless women – you've only got to consider how former British Prime Minister Theresa May and the current First Minister of Scotland, Nicola Sturgeon, have been viewed as a bit "suspect" for being childless, and how each had to "open up" to the press about their struggles to conceive in order to mitigate this somewhat. And it's even harder for childfree-by-choice women, such as the former Prime Minster of Australia, Julia Gillard, who was pilloried in parliament and hounded in the Australian press for being "deliberately barren".

So the harsh truth is that the menopause is a huge loss of status to women, and to childless women even more so. Yes, this might all sound quite primitive, but it's still true.

It is an extraordinary moment when you realise that you've become invisible to men; it's a very strange process. I wrote about it happening to me when I was fifty-two, but I'd been aware of it since my mid-forties. I ruffled quite a few feathers when I wrote about how it was for me, having been an attractive young woman. It turns out you're not allowed to say that – you have to pretend you didn't know you'd been attractive; you can't actually say, in a basic matter-of-fact way, "I was an attractive woman." But it was a fact – just like having green eyes – an accident of birth. And a historical accident, too, that the kind of looks I had as a young woman were what our culture currently deems to be attractive. If I'd been born in a different culture, at a different time, I would have been considered absolutely plain – a tall, skinny, flat-chested freak.

Anyway, I wrote about what that shift was like for me because, when I was younger, I'd found male attention very problematic and it felt delightful that this was passing. It was good not to be hassled all the time, not to be catcalled, and I felt safer as a single woman living alone. But then it moved from that to complete invisibility – I mean, I couldn't even get served in a restaurant anymore! Suddenly, I'm demoted and it's the younger women who are getting served ahead of me by the waiters and they don't even realise they're doing it. So much of this is unconscious and it chips away at your sense of identity, at your sense of value.

When I became postmenopausal, at first I was quite okay with it. I mean, you never quite know which one is your last period, which is weird. But I do remember that a couple of years after that I was cleaning out my bathroom cabinet and found some tampons and I sat on the bathroom floor and wept. I cried for all those years of carrying them around, all the years of hope and all the years of my period arriving and yet again not being pregnant that month – and all the grief too, not just of the menopause but of my entire reproductive history.

Initially, I also felt quite liberated and excited. There's a part of me that had been feeling quite crone-like for some time – maybe because of the dark night of the soul it took for me to get through the grief of childlessness. Yet I'd always looked younger than my age, and I felt excited that I'd now get to live the crone bit on the outside too. But the reality is that, for me, even postmenopausally, the physical symptoms have been pretty rough. Apparently 25 per cent of women sail thorough the menopause without any symptoms – I reckon that's because I've got theirs too!

I calculate that I'm now into my seventeenth year of menopause, counting from that first missed period, and it's still kicking my arse. I've had 50 per cent hair loss in the last three years, which I've found distressing to deal with, and I've had a lot of difficulties getting the balance of my hormones right. A couple of years ago I pretty much bled for nearly a whole year and my menopause specialist said, "Okay, you need more progesterone." My dose was doubled and in a month my entire body was covered in a blanket of soft, dimpled, watery flesh, like you see on very old women. I switched from oral progesterone to a coil but my skin texture didn't recover and so now I've got this dimply, watery flesh all over my body. I've lost muscle mass and a recent bone scan showed that I have osteopenia, which is a worry – I really thought HRT was going to protect me from that. The only upside is that along with my mum's family history of osteoporosis I've also got her oily, olive skin which is a great advantage when you're getting older; I have very few wrinkles. Basically with my clothes on I look fine but with my clothes off I look old.

> But actually, apart from the physical side of the menopause, I love being this age! I love the fierceness.

And that's hard. I aged dramatically, suddenly, and that's been tough to deal with. Maybe the whole crone thing *isn't* going to be a walk in the park...

I still have a lot of sleeping problems and oestrogen helps a little bit, but melatonin is the only thing that works reliably. My hormone balance is changing all the time and that's something that's not well understood: that as our body changes then what needs to be balanced changes too. And so for me it's a constant process of adjusting my hormone levels and finding a practitioner who is skilled and sympathetic in that; they seem to be incredibly rare and, in Ireland, where I now live, there are just a handful of practitioners in the whole country.

But actually, apart from the physical side of the menopause, I love being this age! I love the fierceness. I feel that as a heterosexual woman I gave the years from fifteen to forty-five to men — that I went on some huge reproductive detour and I didn't even get to be a mother! I'm fifty-six now and I'm happy to be free of all that. I presumed I would be single for the rest of my life — I was single through most of my forties apart from a couple of disastrous post-divorce relationships, where I was a complete fruitcake myself. I was an early adopter of internet dating because I've always been an early adopter of new technology, but I really shouldn't have been allowed out — I had such a bad case of babymania and I was still so wounded from the breakdown of my sixteen-year relationship and marriage.

I met my current partner when I was fifty-two. "Current" doesn't feel like the right word — it feels like he's my guy for the rest of my life. And that's lovely because I was single for a long time before meeting him and I'd made my peace with that. I'd embraced it and it turned out that it suited me — I got so much done, it's incredible. I wrote my book, did my psychotherapy training, set up Gateway Women — I did so many things — I was on fire! But it was hard too

– the social isolation can be really tough. When you're middle-aged, single and childless, you really don't get any invitations. I used to joke, "The last invitation I got was for a dental check-up!" but sometimes it really wasn't funny. You drop off the social radar in a truly shocking way and only a few friends survived what I call the hashtag #FriendshipApocalypse of childlessness. Most of them simply sailed off to a country called motherhood, leaving me stranded on the shore without a backward glance. It wasn't malicious, our lives just went in different directions, but whereas their new life came with a whole new social group, mine just emptied out. When this is basically your entire friendship group, as it was with me, that's incredibly painful. It was a big part of the reason I started Gateway Women – to meet new childless friends and I discovered that this experience is very common.

This is actually a beautiful time of life to meet a partner. I remember putting something on Instagram about it, about the joy of finding love in your fifties, when you really know who you are, and you're too damned exhausted by menopause and insomnia to pretend otherwise anyway. It got a lot of likes!

There is a kind of truthfulness that comes with being postmenopausal. You simply don't have the energy or the inclination for a lot of the performative aspects of femininity anymore. It's like, "Take me as I am, and if that's a problem, then that's fine. I can't fake it anymore."

Not only do I not have the energy to fake it anymore, but I also feel that I have an integrity and self-respect now that doesn't allow me to play some of the games I might have played when I was younger, when I thought that's what I had to do in relationships, what you have to do to attract a man. There is a kind of authenticity at this time of life which comes through everything I do.

And that's who my partner met. And he loved it.

For me, the experience of becoming a childless woman massively increased my empathy and opened my eyes to those who are part of any disenfranchised group. The grief of childlessness broke my heart, but it broke it open as well. I suddenly became so much more aware of what it might be like to be a refugee, to be disabled, to be part of the non-dominant ethnicity, to be gay – to be defined by any situation not of your choosing and one that other people use to consider you as "less than". There are so many ways to be othered.

As someone who is white, middle-class passing, reasonably good-looking, well-educated – even though I've had many challenges in my life – I've also had a lot of privilege, unearned privilege. Childlessness stripped me of so much of that – and singleness too – and opened my eyes. It's been a while now and they keep opening further and further – so there is something very powerful about that. And menopause is another one of those portals because the privilege of youth, fertility and attractiveness gets taken away from us too.

Yes, I know that we have the potential to move into a *different* kind of attractiveness, but that takes some getting used to. It's very challenging to talk about because people aren't comfortable with it and tend to push back with comments like, "No, you can still be hot at sixty!"

Well, what if you don't want to be? What about *not* being hot at sixty? What about being comfortable and dumpy? I'm planning to embrace my inner Miss Marple as I get older – I'm going to be that childless old lady in the corner being completely overlooked while in fact I'm one hundred per cent clocking what's going on. It's all about stepping out of that gaze, that male gaze, and embracing something different.

I call the menopause, for childless women, a death you survive. There is a profound grieving process around realising that your genetic line ends with you and it's a great source of shame to a lot of childless women. They feel that they've failed because literally thousands of generations of their ancestors managed to have children, but they haven't. And many often feel that they've let down their own family too, because they haven't given the gift of grandchildren to their parents. Until the menopause comes, quite a few childless women hold on to a last shred of hope for motherhood – even though consciously they know it'd take a miracle. For these women, the menopause is a terrible wake-up call and a painful initiation into the grieving process. I feel so grateful that I'd already come through the worst of my childless grief by the time I had my last period.

One of the really hard things about being a childless woman is that if you try and talk about it, a lot of parents tell you that your childlessness really isn't that bad. They'll say stuff like, "Oh, children aren't all they're cracked up to be," or, "Oh, you've dodged a bullet there," or, "Oh, have one of mine..." Or just, "Aren't you over that yet?" or, "I thought you *chose* not to have children." In the childless community, we call these "bingos" because on a really bad day you can get a full house. Of course, there are people who are childless by choice, or "childfree", a choice I completely respect and admire, but that's only six to ten per cent of women reaching midlife without children. For the rest of us, not having children changes our lives just as much as having children would have done. And for us, the menopause isn't an initiation into our grandmothering years, but learning to live without that experience *too*, both personally and socially.

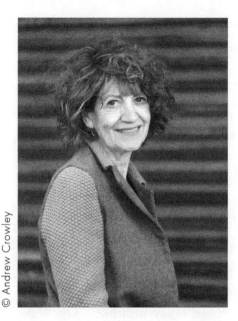

Susie Orbach

Psychoanalyst

"It's not that it bounces you into thinking differently, more that there's something about it that if you don't ignore is profound."

Susie Orbach, 73, is a psychotherapist, psychoanalyst, writer and social critic. She has written widely on women's relationships to their bodies, from her first book, *Fat Is A Feminist Issue*, to *Bodies*, which discusses the ways in which bodies today are becoming sites of display and manufacture rather than a place to live from.

~

I'm seventy-three and the menopause is so not present in my mind now. That is an interesting thing. It's such a dramatic thing at the time but, in a funny way, it's gone when you've passed through it.

The menopause is such a discrete thing because it is the end of something; even if you're not into reproducing, it is the notion of the end of something. When I went through it, I was very aware that it was some kind of marker. What kind of marker it is doesn't become clear to you, but it is a marker. It is the end of a reproductive life, whether you have reproduced or you haven't, whether you've wanted to or not. It's about sexuality, ageing, and a chance to reflect.

I think it's a time when women get a chance to think:

Okay, this is a longer life and what is it that I've learned?

What is it that I need to do?

What is it that I might be stuck in that's imprisoning me?

What's delighting me?

What do I want to open up to?

It's such a powerful physical change for so many women that it can prompt a lot of questions.

Once this is over, have I learned stuff?

Do I have things to offer that I haven't been offering?

Am I bored with what I've been doing?

I think it's that kind of a time.

In terms of symptoms, what I remember is being in meetings and taking off and putting on your jacket all the bloody time. Also I remember the sleep disruptions being horrendous and I think that is why there's a huge industry. You get the women off their Tampax, now let's sell them something else.

It's one of many body industries and it's just getting bigger, especially because of all the forms of HRT, including bioidenticals, and the arguments about how HRT is great for memory and it's great for your bones and it's great for this and that – as though women are always in deficit. We live in a culture where the sell is deficit. Things are sold to us on the notion that there is something missing. And, yes, many women do require medication. But most of the people I know have enough zest once they've gone through the menopause and they do not need it.

I think it is a long damn passage. I don't think it's nothing. And the question around it is: does it allow one to enter into a different kind of way of being in relation to self, in relation to one's sexuality, to reproduction, to the capacity for work and production? It's not that it bounces you into thinking differently, more that there's something about it that if you don't ignore is profound. I do think it is profound.

How we feel about the menopause does link back through to how we've felt about our bodies at all the different stages of our reproductive lives. I think we haven't, in general, brought our daughters up to be excited about periods and so no wonder we haven't prepared ourselves for menopause. We may have taught them it's a curse (I hope not), and then how on earth is anyone prepared for when there is the change and you grow facial hair and lose pubic hair? Or you get hot flushes. I think it's attitudinal to some very large extent, whether we can welcome something that's so damn disruptive, and the menopause is disruptive.

> **Is there something to celebrate in the menopause?**

I didn't take HRT. I'd read the research papers around it. I read the original papers that showed the level of danger and then I read all the propaganda about how that wasn't true and then I read another set of papers. I do feel concerned for women who come off HRT having to go through stuff in their seventies and eighties.

But it's like all issues, for the women for whom it's working that's good for them. I'm not critical. I'm just very aware that in my own group, my friendship group, nobody's taking it.

It's hard for me to know what the menopause was a marker of in my life. Because other life changes happen and then you can graft them on to a thing called menopause. My children were growing up, I'd been in a very long relationship that broke up

– so that's different. You have other griefs and difficult feelings.

I think that marrying a woman could have happened at any point in my life. In the early part of my life I was happily in my relationship and it wasn't on my mind. I don't relate it to menopause at all.

Life isn't static. That is what is so exciting and galling at the same time. It offers you a lot of different opportunities and some of them are full of grief, and some of them are really interesting.

One of the things I did notice during the menopause was how you become socially invisible at a certain point and, more troubling, you didn't know that you counted on the visibility spectrum before. You may not have known that you counted on the male gaze, and then suddenly, it's not there. You realise that's disconcerting. For me it was, "Gosh, I didn't realise how much that was part of it."

Also, during it I felt I very much wanted to do more strength training. I felt like I needed some physical strength and activity. I wasn't a sports person at school at all and I only started aerobic-type exercise when in my mid-thirties before I had kids. So I wasn't somebody for whom sport was a pleasure particularly. But I did start, and did continue to do it. I was very aware that if I wasn't going to take the drugs, I needed to protect my body from osteoporosis.

Interestingly now I am in another phase where strength really is diminishing, and it's shocking. There is no way I can do what I used to do. I'm in a different phase. I think we would have previously called it old age, but I don't feel old. I'm more tired but I'm also still full of energy and I have lots of things I want to do. But, you know, I'm very sympathetic to young people needing all of us to clear off the space and leave it for them.

The first period is a significant moment that could – and I believe should – be celebrated more. It's extraordinary. You are vested with having the capacity to reproduce; whether you do or you don't, it's about having that capacity. I also don't think we celebrate boys' wet dreams either. We don't celebrate anything about this point where we enter into something as a species, as part of the species continuance.

Is there something to celebrate in the menopause? Well, I guess you are free of all that comes with reproductive capacity in theory. You're free of whatever conflicts you might have had about having children, not having children, raising children. I don't know if that's to be celebrated, but I don't think postmenopausal women should be scorned. I think we have lots of interesting things to contribute and say, and we're not really that anxious about fitting in anymore.

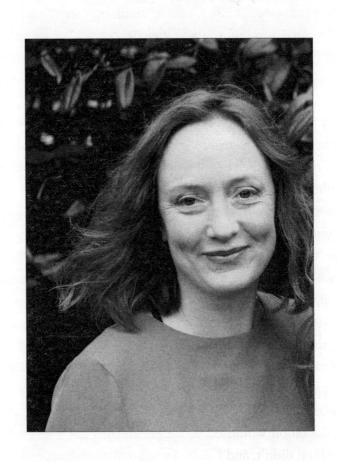

Sharing, the Menopause Revolution Parting Words

Vicky Allan

I literally felt something inside me had died. During the year my periods stopped, an image would keep coming into my mind of a full-skull X-ray I'd had then because of some periodontal treatment. That image, ghostly and menacing, would randomly flash up as a kind of regular memento mori, reminding me not just "you will die", but bits of you, your gums, your jawbone, your ovaries, have already died.

There was a reason for this – it was only partially me being melodramatic about the whole menopause thing. That summer, my brother died, out of the blue, from a pulmonary embolism. I was stricken. In the six months that followed, I possibly had a couple of periods, though to be honest I wasn't keeping count, I wasn't registering. I vaguely remember being on holiday that autumn and taking some tampons in case, almost hopeful for a bleed. Nothing came.

I thought it was shock and stress. I thought once the grief had passed, the blood would come back. But then the months went by and the blood didn't, and I soon started to notice the occasional rush of heat to the head. Was this a hot flush? I was also feeling a death anxiety I'd never had before and which I found hard to pick apart from the menopause symptoms. On a work trip to India, I was going to bed each night and waking up each morning, the only thought repeating in my head, "I am still alive."

That wasn't, as it might sound, a positive thought – rather a recognition of the closeness of death, of my marvel at daily survival. At Christmas I mentioned to my family that I thought I might be menopausal. They asked if I was sure I wasn't pregnant.

I was forty-five and it seemed to me I was way too young for this. I hadn't registered any perimenopause symptoms at all before this sudden full stop of a menopause arrived. I don't think I even knew the word perimenopause existed. The menopause was something that happened to much older women. What I didn't know was that forty-five was just the bottom end of the "normal" menopause range. As I learned while doing the *Still Hot!* interviews, I was not alone in that.

If there's one big theme that comes across in almost all the stories here, it's that somehow the world didn't prepare us for this. It wasn't talked about enough – it was too often jokingly reduced to the single dimension of a comic hot flush. Though in recent years more and more high-profile women have been coming out of the menopausal closet, as Kaye has here, there's still a sense that the Big M is a conversation that occurs mostly below the radar. No one tells you it will be like this. No one really prepares you for it. There has, as Kirsty Wark, put it, been an omertà on menopause.

That omertà is lifting – but only slowly. It's for this reason that we gathered together the many voices in this book – because we recognised that the menopause is not just one story, but many. If we want to make lives better for those going through its many complex variations, we need to share more stories. We need to take the revolution that has already been started in the Menopause Cafés, on daytime television and social media, and spread it wide. We need to make it a conversation that really feels like it is for all – whatever your symptoms, whatever your life experience, your ethnicity, your age, your fertility history, your sexuality, your gender identity.

Because the one-dimensional image we have in our culture is not enough. As psychotherapist Tania Glyde told us, many LGBTQ+ people find the public narrative around the menopause too "hetero-normative (and cisnormative)" and "clichéd". This, as Bunny Cook, trans and nonbinary, observed, can leave those who feel excluded from that narrative, excluded from help.

Many of the voices in this book are high-profile figures already on a mission to end the silence. Others are people with stories that clearly need telling, need broadcasting from the rooftops. I was left moved, tearful, angry, uplifted, in awe – by so many of the interviews.

These are people who shifted my sense of what the menopause is – and reminded me of the way it arrives in so many forms, with such variety of symptoms, knotted up with so many different versions of life experience. Each person goes through it in their own way. That's why we felt this book needed to be written – to express the diversity of menopause – to make it possible that almost anyone might find a bit of themselves between these pages. That said, we know we're still only telling part of the story. The world contains many more than forty-two menopauses.

From the start, I knew a book about the menopause would be not just about the menopause. It would speak of childbirth, not having children, gender identity, femininity, ageing and the thread that weaves back through our lives right to our first period, of shame and confusion. It's about coming out the other end of that fertility journey, whatever we have done with what our unruly bodies have provided us with, and wondering whether you could have lived your life some other way – whether you have even properly engaged with it. In a society without shame around periods and sex might you have had a whole different journey? Could you have had a better relationship to your fertile, or infertile, dangerous, shameful body? Changing how the menopause is seen and felt is inextricably bound up with changing attitudes to fertile-phase female life.

One of the themes that kept cropping up was desire and desirability – whether one is "still hot" – and the title for this book was actually inspired by a joke seen circulating on the internet, the single line, "I'm still hot – it just comes in flushes." The punchline may be about temperature regulation issues, but the joke also acknowledges a need, a pressure, to remain not just sexually active but sexually attractive – to appear both youthful and fertile.

Among those in *Still Hot!*, there were many different thoughts on the question of hotness. While some revelled in their continuing sexiness, others seemed glad to throw off the shackles of desirability, to break out of the cage of sexual objectification. Not everyone had enjoyed the expectations that exist around women in their fertile years. As Jody Day puts it, "What about *not* being hot at sixty? What about being comfortable and dumpy? I'm planning to embrace my inner Miss Marple as I get older."

In doing these interviews I came to appreciate that how we feel about the menopause varies almost as much as the symptoms. It depends on our cultural experience, our life events, our menstrual cycle history and many other factors. It can even be about when it happens. I was one of those who hadn't seen it coming – and wasn't ready for it. I felt that something suddenly had been stolen from me. There was none of that relief at the end of periods – only a desire to have them back.

It wasn't so much that I wanted anything more of my fertility, wanted another baby – I was already in my mid-forties and felt blessed to have two lovely sons – but, like the loss of my brother, this was a death too early, too soon, too sudden, too unexpected, too uncontemplated. I'd had almost as little thought of the approach of my menopause as I had the possibility of the death of my brother.

But that shock pales by comparison with those who were thrown it much earlier. I was tear-struck talking with those who took that blow in their thirties. For Michelle Heaton, Sahira Ahmad Belcher and Andrea Macfarlane, the journey was made still lonelier by the fact that they were embarking on it outside their peer group, and at an age when the assumption is that they might still be fertile, and when they might even have hoped of another child.

And I heard of how even if menopause arrives, as if on schedule, between forty-five and fifty-five, it can still deliver a blow of grief, particularly if like Yvonne John, Jody Day and Paulette Edwards, it brings a brutal finality to unwanted childlessness. Its message of loss is immense.

One of the things that struck me was how the menopause doesn't exist on its own. It is not a set of standalone symptoms. Our experience of it, and even our hormonal balance as we go through it, is affected by what goes on in our lives. As Nimmy March put it, the menopause gets "woven through" our life events. It can be there when, like Anthea Turner, we are divorcing, or like Danusia Malina-Derben we have had a set of triplets late in our forties, or like Alison Martin-Campbell we are first supporting our elderly parents, and later mourning their deaths.

It affects our work, our play, our relationships. Many in this book spoke of being unable to pick apart what caused what, what exacerbated what, what was age, what was menopause, what was life. Myself, I don't know if the wave of anxiety and insomnia I had in my mid-forties, and always thought of as "just grief", had been destined by my ovaries and stirred up by my hormones, or if the stress of loss charged up my menopause, even brought it on early. I remember asking Google whether grief can "cause" the menopause.

The menopause can bring a revelation around our perceptions of what even we are. Faced with this hormonal cataclysm, we can start to wonder how much of what we feel, what we consider our identity, has been defined by the interactions of our reproductive hormones. When they fade away, who are we? And who really were we, in the throes of that cycle?

The stories that hit me most are the ones that touched on some of the biggest taboos. We may all be up for talking about rage and brain fog, but are we really up for a frank discussion about sex post-menopause? It was almost a relief to hear Tracey Cox's admission that even she, highly sexed as she once was, has felt her libido drop through the floor. Jane Lewis's excruciating description of her own vaginal atrophy, and what she understands of the genito-urinary problems in care homes, filled me with horror and made me want to start a conversation about this with almost every older woman I know.

All this can sound a bit depressing. I have to admit I was filled with doom and menopause gloom when I started, mid-Covid lock-down, the interviews for this book. I felt my life was on the slide. I'd squandered opportunities. But what I noticed was that almost every interview I did lifted my mood.

The arrival of the menopause is like slowly turning the Death card in the Tarot deck. The first feeling is dread, but then it dawns that this could be a new beginning, the third act, as much about fresh life as its ending. As some women have put it here, menopause can be a superpower. It can be the thing that tips us over from ticking along into being life-seekers. We see that again and again in these stories. Faced with anxiety, sleeplessness, lack of control, Louise Minchin takes up triathlon, Erica Clarkson starts running her Meno Ultras, Trinny Woodall reinvents herself as a makeup entrepreneur, Marie Louise Cochrane hosts storytelling events around sex.

More than that, for almost everyone in *Still Hot!*, the menopause really is a transition from one self to another – it's a journey. Sharon

Blackie spoke eloquently about where it can take us, what gets burned away, what we shed on the passage to elderhood and how we can use this time to look inwards, to cultivate wisdom, to draw on our experience.

All of us here have in some way left our old selves behind. Already I feel I almost don't quite remember my pre-menopause self. My brother's death and the start of my menopause are like a black line dividing parts of my life. The before seems like some hazy other self – still fertile, still bleeding, still sleeping . . . I sometimes wonder who she was. The now seems like a fog I am still navigating my way through.

One of the questions I had for myself was whether I wanted to go on HRT. I had told myself I was at peace with my symptoms – that they weren't that bad. But then I listened to women like Erica Clarkson or Louise Minchin telling me they would take HRT till they died, and I would crave some of that energy, that special drive they had. Am I really at peace? I began to wonder. Or just coping? Could things be better?

But at the same time, I was interviewing other women with different answers to the challenge of the menopause, who had their own version of that drive and energy. I loved Sharon Blackie's idea of "hagitude". Chatting with her, I found all I wanted was some of that hag power, that incandescence – and it struck me there was something compelling here that wasn't about pills or gels or no pills, but about women of this age and their almost electric charge.

The menopause can all too easily divide us, as so many experiences in women's lives can. Are you a breast- or a bottle-feeder? Natural birth or caesarean? HRT or toughing it out to become a wise old crone? One of the conclusions I came to is that it's possible to do both. I'm still not yet on HRT, but I'm seriously considering it. Every person here is on a journey, making a transition, learning and becoming something they weren't before their hormones untethered them and sent them, reeling, through this change, and made them someone they weren't before. Sharing stories can help break down divisions – it can help us see what we have in common in the often-difficult passage of the menopause. It can help us understand that it's not HRT versus wise woman.

Most of the big feminist revolutions of recent times have involved sharing stories. We have seen the impact of MeToo, the power of *Know My Name*, as well as the fight against period poverty and the lifting of period shame through story-sharing. The menopause needs its own movement. It already has one, burgeoning and growing, developed by some of the voices here, as well as countless others outside this book. Almost a twin to the movement around period shame and period poverty, it's a reminder that changing attitudes to the menopause is an important element in changing attitudes to women, gender and bodies, in general.

We hope these stories will make you go out and share your own, or, even if you're not experiencing the menopause yourself, join the conversation. For this hormonal upheaval is not something just experienced by women on their own, but by all those around them, by all of society. It is something that all of us who float in this human sea of clashing hormones – of puberty, andropause, pregnancy, post-partum – are touched by in some way. Let's not let it pass silently. Let's roar the M-word from the rooftops. Let's overshare.

Resources & Reading

There are more and more sites, organisations and books to turn to if you're struggling with your menopause, wondering how best to handle it, wanting some hard facts, or simply looking for some support and solidarity. We list some here.

CUTIC.CO.UK – It's not purely about the menopause, but the site of the Chronic Urinary Tract Infection Campaign is an excellent source of information for those going through the infections so often associated with hormonal change, with an important mission to raise awareness.

DAISYNETWORK.ORG – For those lonely and isolated with premature ovarian failure/primary ovarian insufficiency (early menopause), this charity is a vital source of support and information.

GATEWAY-WOMEN.COM – The revolutionary support network for women "united by and beyond childlessness", set up by Jody Day. It's an online community, global friendship network and provider of videos, podcasts and workshops.

HYPERHIDROSISUK.ORG – There's a term for the disorder of excessive sweating – one sometimes associated with the menopause – and it's hyperhidrosis. For those who suffer it, the International Hyperhidrosis Society is a source of support and information.

MEGSMENOPAUSE.COM – Information resource, shop and events platform, all brought together by Meg Matthews, icon of the Britpop era. When Meg turned fifty and started experiencing menopause symptoms, she was shocked at the lack of support and understanding and made it her mission "to break the stigma".

MENOPAUSECAFE.NET – There are others out there like you and wouldn't it be wonderful to chat over a cuppa? This genius idea started by Rachel Weiss, in Perth, and based on the Death Café model, is spreading across the world and if there's not a menopause café near you, you can always start one.

MENOPAUSEDOCTOR.CO.UK – By Dr Louise Newson, providing information on HRT and alternatives, plus many downloadable booklets. There's a downloadable app, balance, which provides free evidence-based information, a health journal and community features.

MENOPAUSEMATTERS.CO.UK – Set up by Dr Heather Currie in 2002 to provide support and information so that "all women are able to make informed decisions about management of their menopause". Everything from symptoms to HRT and lifestyle advice. Also provides an email consultation service and a forum where you can share and discuss with others.

MENOPAUSESUPPORT.CO.UK – Diane Danzebrink had to have a total hysterectomy, including removal of both ovaries, putting her into immediate surgical menopause. The dark place she found herself in, with no support and counselling, drove her to campaign for menopause awareness. Support her campaign and find a link to her #MakeMenopauseMatter petition.

MYMENOPAUSALVAGINA.CO.UK — This website promoting the Jane Lewis book, *Me & My Menopausal Vagina*, is a brilliant source of information relating to vaginal atrophy and includes downloadable leaflets and helpful links, as well as Jane's blog.

SAMARITANS.ORG — It's not uncommon to have suicidal thoughts during the menopause. If you have them, there is always someone you can talk to. Call the Samaritans for free on 116 123.

WWW.NHS.UK/CONDITIONS/MENOPAUSE/ — An overview of menopause symptoms and the treatments available. As the site recommends, your GP is the best first port of call if your symptoms are troubling you.

~

Sam Baker, *The Shift: How I (lost and) found myself after 40 — and you can too*, Hachette (2020)

Sharon Blackie, *If Women Rose Rooted: A Life-changing Journey to Authenticity and Belonging*, September Publishing (2016)

Tracey Cox, *Great Sex Starts at 50: How to age-proof your libido*, Murdoch Books (2020)

Christa D'Souza, *Hot Topic: A life-changing look at the Change of Life*, Short Books (2016)

Liz Earle, *The Good Menopause Guide*, Orion (2018)

Jenny Eclair, *Older and Wider: A Survivor's Guide to the Menopause*, Quercus (2020)

Helen FitzGerald, *Worst Case Scenario*, Orenda (2019)

Louise Foxcroft, *Hot Flushes, Cold Science: A History of the Modern Menopause*, Granta (2010)

Andrea Glover, *The Perimenopause Handbook: What Every Women Needs to Know About the Transition from Perimenopause into Menopause*, New Leaf Media (2020)

Germaine Greer, *The Change: Women, Aging and the Menopause*, Hamish Hamilton (1991)

Michelle Heaton, *Hot Flush: Menopause, Motherhood and Me*, Michael O'Mara (2018)

Dr Philippa Kaye, *The M Word: Everything You Need to Know About the Menopause*, Vie (2020)

Andrea McLean, *Confessions of a Menopausal Woman: Everything you want to know but are too afraid to ask . . .*, Bantam (2018)

Jenni Murray, *Is It Me Or Is It Hot In Here?: A Modern Woman's Guide to the Menopause*, Vermillion (2003)

Dr Louise Newson, *Menopause: All you need to know in one concise manual*, J H Haynes & Co Ltd (2019)

Christiane Northrup, MD, *The Wisdom of Menopause: Creating Physical and Emotional Health During the Change*, Random House (2012)

Penny Pepper, *Desires Reborn*, Bejamo (2003)

Miranda Sawyer, *Out Of Time: midlife, if you still think you're young*, HarperCollins (2016)

Gail Sheehy, *The Silent Passage: Menopause*, Random House (1991)

Darcey Steinke, *Flash Count Diary: A New Story About the Menopause*, Canongate (2019)

Menopause Bingo

Since BBC presenter Louise Minchin mentioned her habit of playing Menopause Bingo with her friends, we haven't been able to resist it either. This is the full list of thirty-four symptoms. Have a go yourself. But here's hoping you don't get the full house.

1. Hot flushes
2. Night sweats
3. Irregular periods
4. Mood swings
5. Vaginal dryness
6. Decreased libido
7. Headaches
8. Breast soreness
9. Burning mouth
10. Joint pain
11. Digestive problems
12. Electric shocks
13. Muscle tension
14. Gum problems
15. Tingling extremities
16. Itchy skin
17. Fatigue
18. Anxiety
19. Disrupted sleep
20. Hair loss
21. Memory lapses
22. Difficulty concentrating
23. Weight gain
24. Dizzy spells
25. Bloating
26. Stress incontinence
27. Brittle nails
28. Allergies
29. Irregular heartbeat
30. Body odour
31. Irritability
32. Depression
33. Panic disorder
34. Osteoporosis

Thanks

With grateful thanks to all of our frank and fearless contributors for collectively giving us a full 360-degree menopause. You pave the way for others. To our mums, Cathie Adams (aka Mrs A. and menopause-denier-in-chief), and Sylvia Allan, always up for a chat about any hot topic. And also to the whole team at Black & White, especially Ali McBride, who dreamed up this scheme, and Emma Hargrave, ever wise, through all our fog, rage, lows and sparks of inspiration.